THE COMPLETE IDIOT'S GUIDE® TO

Your True Age

by Judith Partnow Hyman, Ph.D., and Elaine Bernstein Partnow

ALPHA

A member of Penguin Group (USA) Inc.

To our husbands, Turner Browne and Herbert Hyman, D.D.S. Their companionship, intelligence, and wholehearted support in all we do has buoyed us and helped us achieve mature AQs.

ALPHA BOOKS

Published by the Penguin Group

Penguin Group (USA) Inc., 375 Hudson Street, New York, New York 10014, USA

Penguin Group (Canada), 90 Eglinton Avenue East, Suite 700, Toronto, Ontario M4P 2Y3, Canada (a division of Pearson Penguin Canada Inc.)

Penguin Books Ltd., 80 Strand, London WC2R 0RL, England

Penguin Ireland, 25 St. Stephen's Green, Dublin 2, Ireland (a division of Penguin Books Ltd.)

Penguin Group (Australia), 250 Camberwell Road, Camberwell, Victoria 3124, Australia (a division of Pearson Australia Group Pty. Ltd.)

Penguin Books India Pvt. Ltd., 11 Community Centre, Panchsheel Park, New Delhi—110 017, India

Penguin Group (NZ), 67 Apollo Drive, Rosedale, North Shore, Auckland 1311, New Zealand (a division of Pearson New Zealand Ltd.)

Penguin Books (South Africa) (Pty.) Ltd., 24 Sturdee Avenue, Rosebank, Johannesburg 2196, South Africa

Penguin Books Ltd., Registered Offices: 80 Strand, London WC2R 0RL, England

Copyright © 2008 by Elaine Bernstein Partnow and Judith Partnow Hyman, Ph.D.

International Standard Book Number: 978-1-59257-822-1
Library of Congress Catalog Card Number: 2008927335

10 09 08   8 7 6 5 4 3 2 1

Interpretation of the printing code: The rightmost number of the first series of numbers is the year of the book's printing; the rightmost number of the second series of numbers is the number of the book's printing. For example, a printing code of 08-1 shows that the first printing occurred in 2008.

Printed in the United States of America

Note: This publication contains the opinions and ideas of its authors. It is intended to provide helpful and informative material on the subject matter covered. It is sold with the understanding that the authors and publisher are not engaged in rendering professional services in the book. If the reader requires personal assistance or advice, a competent professional should be consulted.

The authors and publisher specifically disclaim any responsibility for any liability, loss, or risk, personal or otherwise, which is incurred as a consequence, directly or indirectly, of the use and application of any of the contents of this book.

Most Alpha books are available at special quantity discounts for bulk purchases for sales promotions, premiums, fund-raising, or educational use. Special books, or book excerpts, can also be created to fit specific needs.

For details, write: Special Markets, Alpha Books, 375 Hudson Street, New York, NY 10014.

Publisher: *Marie Butler-Knight*
Editorial Director: *Mike Sanders*
Senior Managing Editor: *Billy Fields*
Acquisitions Editor: *Michele Wells*
Development Editor: *Jennifer Moore*
Production Editor: *Kayla Dugger*

Copy Editor: *Jan Zoya*
Cartoonist: *Steve Barr*
Cover Designer: *Bill Thomas*
Book Designers: *Trina Wurst, Kurt Owens*
Indexer: *Brad Herriman*
Layout: *Chad Dressler*
Proofreader: *Laura Caddell*

Contents at a Glance

Contents

Introduction

Youth is as much a state of mind as it is a time and place in life. Just as in our later years we can be very young in some things, so during our so-called "youth" we may be very old in others.

The Complete Idiot's Guide to Your True Age is predicated on the theory that within each of us exists many ages; we call these age quotients. The book is designed to help you find out just what your personal age quotients are.

Thirteen Candles

In 1983 Howard Gardner introduced the world to his theory of multiple intelligences in his seminal book, *Frames of Mind*. Each of us, he theorized, possesses varying capabilities and potential in at least six areas: linguistic, musical, logical-mathematical, spatial, bodily kinesthetic, and personal. The traditional attitude about intelligence, with tests to measure one's IQ, did not, Gardner argued, take into account these other intelligences. Since that time, others who support Gardner's view have added two more intelligences: naturalistic-nature intelligence and, instead of personal intelligence, interpersonal intelligence and intrapersonal intelligence (the former being how well you know yourself and the latter how well you know and understand others).

Eight intelligences. So why should we be stuck with only one age?

A lemon tree, like everything else, has a chronological age. But what are the ages of the lemons it bears? Each has its season, and within that, its own age. So it is with us. The fruits we bear during infancy are quite different from those of adolescence. The varying seasons of early, middle, and late adulthood all blossom anew, bearing fresh fruit, green fruit that needs ripening.

Each cell in your body has its own age. Some renew themselves every few days, while others over a period of several years. How old are your kidneys, your fingernails, your skin, your hair? These changes are part of a deterioration process as well as a constant rebirth. It is a dialectic of life, as changing and as constant as the sea.

As we attain experience, develop skills, and grow our perceptions, our comprehension of the world around us changes. Old value systems may drop away much as ripe fruit drops from the branch, making room for the flowering and inevitable new growth. Examine your work ethic, your spiritual goals, and the values you place on family, friends, possessions, hobbies. Are they the same now as they were 20, even 10 years ago? Probably not. So how "old" are they?

You may wonder why we chose a lemon tree to illustrate our point. Why not peaches or apples? Who wants to be compared to a lemon? In America, aging is like a lemon—a bitter fruit. But by adding a little sweetener and plenty of fresh water, you can make a delightfully refreshing lemonade. Or by adding a little salt and tequila, you've got yourself the ingredients for a rip-roaring fun time. Rather than being sour, a lemon—like age—can be part of the seasoning of life: natural, cleansing, strengthening, enjoyable, intoxicating. It can be mixed and enjoyed by all ages, for all ages.

Each chapter begins with a series of questions to help establish your age quotient (AQ) for that category. Some of you may be shocked to find you have an elevated age in one section and a juvenile age in another. Remember, age has a different meaning for each category. When dealing with fitness or medical age, clearly a youthful age quotient is desirable; when dealing with work age, it is not (you don't still want to be delivering newspapers on your bicycle when you're 38, do you?).

If one of the figures in your age profile looks out of whack with the others, look back at the questions heading that chapter and see if one of them doesn't pinpoint a particular area you might want to reappraise or examine.

Some age quotients will be quite a bit higher than your actual age. Are you thinking, "Oh, gee, that's bad"? Guess again. Maturity, wisdom, self-knowledge—these are some of the rewards a person earns from putting in some time on this good Earth. Possession of these traits will boost several of your AQs, as would a stable home life and a solid self-image.

If you have a good position in society, economic security, and are in stride with the times, it is likely that your AQs in these areas will be higher than your chronological age. If your AQs in these areas are low, use that as a clue to re-examine your work possibilities or your awareness of the world around you.

The quizzes are not scientific examinations of aging. Nor do they attempt to fit you into a mold. What they do offer is a self-appraisal guide aimed at raising your age consciousness. There is no set scale by which to measure your—or anyone's —age quotients. Your own good judgment and earnestness in learning about yourself are the basic prerequisites that can turn this book into a helpful tool.

When you've completed all the quizzes and done the scoring, with a simple formula, you can add up all your age quotients plus your chronological age to discover your true age.

How This Book Is Organized

We've divided this book into the following parts:

Part 1, "Explanations," introduces you to the concept of age quotients, examining the very essence of age itself. There's a brief review of the several ingredients of longevity. And there's a thorough explanation of the quizzes and how to tabulate your age quotients.

Part 2, "Physical Age Quotients," helps you ascertain your four physical age quotients: medical, physical fitness, sexuality, and brain fitness (yes, brain fitness: you don't want your brain to start sagging, do you?). Unless you're in your 20s, you're going to hope for an AQ younger than your years, right? Well, yes—and no. You'll have to take the tests, read the chapters, and see.

Part 3, "Your Inner Workings," deals with a little mystery. We start with your own self-image (which has an impact on every single aspect of your age quotients) and move on to your spiritual age quotient, which has nothing to do with whether or not you're active in a church, mosque, or synagogue. It deals with your inner spiritual life. Last, we help you to establish your future age quotient: how you approach, prepare for, and adapt to this quickly changing world.

Part 4, "The World Around You," presents the last six age quotient categories. They all deal with relationships. If you have a significant other, you'll take the quiz for that chapter; if you live alone, the singleness chapter is for you, although you may have a special friend and therefore want to take the significant other quiz as well. Everyone will want to discover his true age with family, friends, finances, and the community at large. Generally speaking, age quotients close to your own age, give or take a few years, are the norm in this section. But there are some exceptions.

Helpful Additions

To enhance your reading pleasure, we have generously sprinkled the text with sidebars—boxes of interesting, helpful, and entertaining information.

Optimize Your AQ _____

Tips and suggestions to aid you in establishing habits and attitudes that lead to optimizing your true age.

def•i•ni•tion _____

Here you'll find definitions of terms you might not be familiar with.

Birthday Blahs _____

Take good care of yourself by heeding these words of caution.

How Many Candles? _____

Here you'll find mini-profiles of people who have taken the same quizzes you're about to. After reading the thumbnail sketch, you may be surprised to learn these people's true ages and their chronological ages.

Wisdom of the Ages _____

Brief vignettes to entertain and amuse you while elucidating true age attitudes.

Acknowledgments

We would like to thank all those who gave of their time and thoughtfulness in taking our preliminary quizzes, which provided us with material for analyses and the mini-profiles. Several friends took extra time to help out: Herb Hyman, D.D.S., who double-checked the accuracy of medical terms and explanations; Sue Witkovsky, Bette Glenn, and Susan Partnow for feedback on the quizzes; Del Jones for information on sage-ing circles; Mary Ann Whiteman for her detailed commentary on singleness, and Glynn Marsh Allen. We're also very appreciative of the supportive staff at Alpha Books: Michele Wells, who encouraged us to "run with the ball" on our theory of age quotients; Kayla Dugger, who helped keep us on track; and both Jennifer Moore and Jan Zoya, whose conscientious editing helped clarify and improve our work. We'd also like to thank our agents, Sheree Bykofsky and Janet Rosen, for all they do (special thanks to Janet for providing some fun story material).

Trademarks

All terms mentioned in this book that are known to be or are suspected of being trademarks or service marks have been appropriately capitalized. Alpha Books and Penguin Group (USA) Inc. cannot attest to the accuracy of this information. Use of a term in this book should not be regarded as affecting the validity of any trademark or service mark.

Part 1

Explanations

There's been a lot of talk in the media about people's "true" or "real" age lately. Not sure what people are referring to by these terms? The following chapters help you make sense of these concepts, and explain how you can go about calculating your true age, as distinguished from your chronological age.

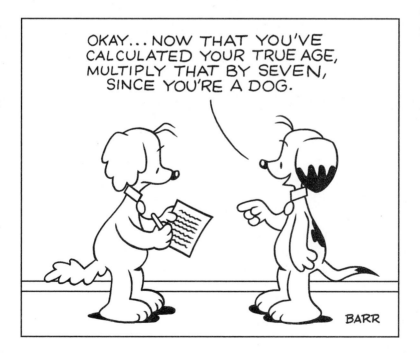

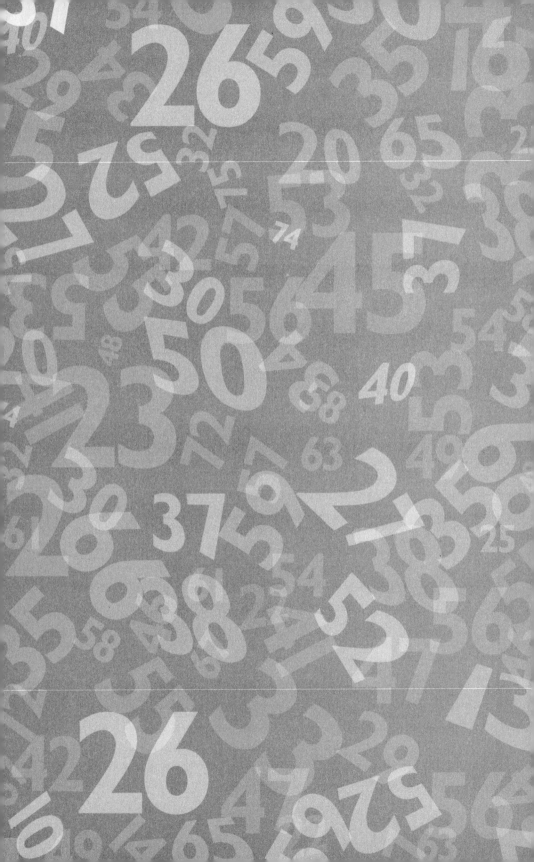

Chapter 1

What Is an "Age Quotient"?

In This Chapter

- ◆ Finding out what an age quotient is
- ◆ Exploring the relativity of age
- ◆ Discovering what is and is not natural to aging
- ◆ Considering the influence of the media on age and aging
- ◆ Learning how language affects age and aging

Few people like to answer the question, "How old are you?" It pins you to a spot, often a very narrow one, that says little about who you are, how you are, what you are, and what you think. Wouldn't you rather answer that question with, "That all depends. Are you talking about my family age, my social age, or my spiritual age? They're all different, you know."

What Is Age?

How many times have you heard an exchange like this: "Your daughter is darling, truly an amazing child. How old is she?" "Oh. She's 7 going on 35." Or what about this one: "Your husband is such a football enthusiast. I can't believe he still plays tackle with your boys." "Oh yes, my husband is 48 going on 16." Such dialogues may evoke laughter, a sagacious nodding of the head, or eyes rolling heavenward. Whatever your response, what such comments point out is that chronological age is just the tip of the iceberg. It doesn't begin to reveal what's underneath.

When your birthday rolls around, you may enjoy celebrating it or you may find it depressing. But what is its real significance? It measures only that you've lived another 365 days. Age is a subjective experience. Some days fly by while others never seem to end. And the measure of a day is relative to the total number of days in your life. One day is a much greater chunk of time in the life of a boy of 8 than it is in the life of a 38-year-old.

Chronological age is an imposition from the objective world, one that attempts to fit everyone into the same frame of reference. But individuals are unique, possessing several frames of reference, several "measurements of time." In this book, we call these age quotients, or AQs for short.

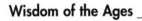

Wisdom of the Ages

Einstein proved that time and space can no longer be measured in terms of absolutes, but only in terms of an object's frame of reference. The same must be true with age, for what is age but time?

The Journey of Aging

Aging is a unique journey that can be observed with as much pleasure and amazement in childhood as during the adult years. Just as children have much to learn from their adult role models, so adults have much to learn from youngsters. Children's lack of self-consciousness, their wide-eyed wonder and eagerness to learn, their absolute need to explore and discover—these are yours for the recapturing.

In his book *The Role of the Aged in Primitive Society*, Leo Simmons recounts a dialogue between some elders of the African Akamba tribe and one of the younger tribesmen who had just returned from a trip abroad. Upon hearing the younger man's account of the adventure, two of the elders responded. "Young man," said one, "if you speak the truth, you are old. You have seen much; we are but children." The second aged man, a chief, added, "Young man, we thank you for your news. You have made us older than we were, but you are older still, for you have seen with your eyes, what we only hear with our ears."

These people recognized the value of direct experience, and knew that time is the corral into which each experience may be gathered. In their slower-moving society, the eyewitness reports of the many things their younger clansman had seen and done in the fast-paced world outside their village classified him as one who had spent much time in the world. Perhaps they somehow saw that he'd managed to compress time, thus becoming older than they—something reminiscent of Einstein's general theory of relativity: time and space can no longer be measured in terms of absolutes, but only in terms of an object's frame of reference. When it comes to age, the frame of reference of a child is entirely different than that of an adult, and the frame of reference for a young adult is entirely different than it is for elders.

As life expectancy increases, it's important to learn to accept the reality that everyone is both young and old at the same time. Children can be very old in their youth, just as elders who have maintained their health and vigor seem to have an agelessness in the very lines on their faces.

The Changes Age Brings

Once you're past the teen years, the changes brought about by aging are gradual and subtle. There is continued growth and development of your body and brain in young adulthood, but nothing quite so dramatic as in your earlier years. As you move toward what is usually termed middle age, you may witness further changes—graying or loss of hair, crow's-feet and laugh lines, sagging muscle tone, a thicker frame. If you are healthy, you will find that the added patience and diligence that comes with maturity will more than compensate for any physical slowing down, resulting in increased accuracy. Learning skills are honed. To top it off, maturity acts to sort out the emotional confusion so often experienced in youth.

Over 30 years ago, studies of infants, youths, and the elderly abounded, but nothing for those in between. *Gerontologists* tended to ignore the stretch of time between the ages of 25 and 65. Why? Perhaps because the changes that take place during adulthood are so subtle, they are difficult to measure and observe. But new technology and advanced science has changed all that.

def•i•ni•tion

A **gerontologist** is a scientist who studies the biological, psychological, and sociological phenomena associated with aging and old age.

More and more scientists have begun to explore the middle years. The baby boomer population has altered the concept of what was once termed "old age": 60 has replaced 40 as the new middle age. Middle-agers hold more social roles than any other age group—worker, parent, spouse, hobbyist, sports enthusiast, traveler, student, theatergoer, sibling, daughter/son, grandparent, caretaker, consumer, car owner, property holder, investor, and so on. In terms of upholding the economy, no other group is as influential.

But there is a lot of age prejudice in society, which has tended to fixate on an ideal of youth despite the fact that we are "witnessing the graying and not the greening of America," as renowned sociologist Amitai Etzioni put it. The U.S. Census Bureau (USCB) shows that by 2029, all of the baby boomers (those born between 1946 and 1964) will be 65 years and over.

Wisdom of the Ages

In this country, some people start being miserable about growing old while they are still young.

—Margaret Mead

As Americans get healthier and life spans increase, the whole concept of age groups changes. "Middle age is what your parents are," a friend once said. Indeed, a sliding scale is the only practical tool for measuring age.

Natural Aging

Despite fears to the contrary, physical collapse is not a mandate of aging. It can occur at any time along the chronological scale. Canadian endocrinologist Dr. Hans Selye, whose seminal works brought light to bear on the diseases caused by stress, wrote in *The Stress of Life:* "Among my autopsies (and I have performed quite a few), I have never seen a man who died of old age .... True physiological aging is not determined by the time elapsed since birth, but by the total amount of wear and tear to which the body has been exposed." In Chapters 3 through 6, we discuss your medical, physical fitness, sexuality, and brain fitness age quotients (or AQs, as we refer to them). There you will see that, indeed, "one may be much more senile in body and mind, and much closer to the grave, at 40 than another person at 60."

How Many Candles?

A divorced retiree, this New Yorker rents an apartment where he lives on a modest income. His grown children have provided him with two grandchildren. He has a sister. Although he was born Jewish, he has no religious affiliation, yet his spiritual life is on firm ground (AQ 65). He drinks moderately and quit smoking more than five years ago. Despite being a little bit overweight, he's careful about having his annual checkups (medical AQ 20), and he exercises four to five times a week (physical fitness AQ 35). Politically, he's very liberal, with a keen interest in current affairs as well as the arts. He votes in all elections and makes contributions, but is not at all involved in the life of his community (AQ 46). While he enjoys living alone, he'd be open to a relationship, if he could only meet someone (AQ 28). The hardest part of being single for him is the lack of sex; he has a mature sexuality AQ of 42.

His true age is 42. His chronological age: 77! If this conscientious fellow became more involved in community affairs, he'd be more likely to meet someone with whom he could have a relationship, which would both raise his community AQ and lower his sexuality AQ.

Society seems to have a keener awareness of body age than of intellectual age. In fact, throughout modern history, the body has been so all-important that even in death it consumes a great deal of industry and expense. Whereas much ado over the body may add to your enjoyment of life and to your life span, not enough ado over other aspects of aging may counter that effort.

The four physical age quotients—medical, physical fitness, sexuality, and brain fitness—lay the foundation for a healthy, fulfilling life. The inner age quotients—self-image, spiritual, future—offer strengths of a different kind: adaptability, resilience, self-knowledge, self-confidence, and faith. Without strength in these areas, the age quotients in the outer world—relationships with family, significant others, friends, and the workplace—would have far less meaning in our lives.

The Media and the Mess of Age

If you looked at societies as having age quotients, you'd have to admit that America's is quite juvenile. America is a nation of youth worshippers. About 560 times a day, youth is hawked from magazines, blaring radios and TVs, and roadside billboards. The Internet bombards users with ads for eliminating cellulite and wrinkles, flattening stomachs, and increasing the size of breasts and penises. If you're like most people, these messages ring in your ears and send shivers down your spine.

Wisdom of the Ages

A man, as he manages himself, may die old at 30 or young at 80.

—Shaker Proverb

It's essential to develop some psychic armor to protect yourself from this onslaught, so that your self-image becomes a reflection of what you think of yourself, not some manufactured image. Think of it as a sort of "ageist meter" that raises your consciousness so you won't be vulnerable to these attacks on your self-image.

How? Here's one way: pick up a magazine, any magazine. Look at the ads. The women depicted are, almost without exception, extremely attractive, beautifully dressed (or undressed), and slender. If they are older women, they seem unaffected by age. None of the men have pot bellies, all are very dashing, and most are under 40. Even the ads in *AARP, the Magazine* show adults in their 30s, 40s, and 50s, all very trim and attractive and with dashingly lined faces.

The situation is much the same on television shows and commercials. As you raise your consciousness, you will make healthier choices in what you watch and what you read.

The American public is getting older. Advertisers will have to stop catering to the young. But "engineered fads," as futurist Alvin Toffler calls them, are nothing new to the advertising industry. Without a doubt, as soon as big business orders it, advertisers will sell middle age just as they have sold youth. Already Clairol has a line of varying shades of gray dyes to "correct" naturally gray hair: it is now chic to be gray. Age can be made to sell.

But while science and medicine strive to help us live longer, the media, by and large, still strives to make us obsolete at younger and younger ages. However, with your ageist meter in full swing, you will soon recognize whether *you* are being recognized or dissed!

You can use your consumer power to boycott products that tout ageist messages; you can register your complaints with the folks on Madison Avenue. You can help straighten out the "mess of age" in the media.

The Language of Age

More than anything else, language shapes and molds the most powerful, detailed pictures you have of the world around you and of yourself. Whether you read a book or a blog, watch a movie, or listen to the radio, language impacts you. In conversations with your boss, clients, and friends; dialogues between teacher and students; parents and children; husband and wife; patient and doctor, language impacts you. Whether you're giving instructions to employees or merchants, or making pleas to policemen, politicians, or petty thieves, language impacts you.

Each time a word or a series of words forms in your brain, a biochemical reaction occurs: however subtly, you are physically and mentally changed.

Some words disappear (no one uses "avaricious" anymore), new words are invented (whoever heard of a "blog" 15 years ago?), and many words change their meaning (think of the word "gay"). But some words never

Wisdom of the Ages

Age is a state of mind—or mindlessness.
—Garson Kanin

change. Like the word "old." Even without expression, it seems negative. It calls to mind something falling apart, something useless, decrepit, to be thrown away. Yet of the eight definitions of the word "old" in the *American Heritage Dictionary*, "worn out" is way down the line: (1) having lived or existed for a relatively long time; *far advanced* (our emphasis) in years of life. (2) made long ago; ancient. (3) characteristic of an aged person. (4) *Mature; sensible* (again our emphasis). (5) having a specific age: "she was two years old." (6) of an earlier time: "his old classmates." (7) worn out.

Considering this, why should the word "old" always seem to connote stodginess, slowing down, rigidity, and decrepitude? Why not mature, advanced in life, cherished?

Ageism in language can be very subtle, and it may not be as immediately apparent as racist or sexist terms. Like its counterparts, however, it is equally necessary to rid language of ageist expressions.

Optimize Your AQ

Even doctors make ageist assumptions: An older man was suffering from severe pain in one of his knees when he went to see his physician. The doctor probed and pinched, took X-rays, but could find nothing wrong. "You'll just have to grin and bear it," he told his patient. "These things happen when we get older." "Just a darn minute there," the old man replied. "What do you mean, 'these things happen'? My other knee is doing just fine, and it's the same age as the one that hurts!"

Nonageist Terminology

Years ago, the droll and notable columnist Jack Smith took up the problem of age and language. He offered a new word to the nomenclature of gerontology—*genarian,* a kind of shortcut for *sexagenarian, septuagenarian, octogenarian, nonagenarian,* and *centenarian.* Genarian would be a general term for all those over 60, or past midlife.

Perhaps our lives could simply be divided into thirds: from birth to 30 (youth); from 30 to 60 (adults); over 60 (generians). Anyone or anything showing discrimination toward any of these age groups would be guilty of ageism. And those terrified of moving from one age to the next, a common fear generated by the rampant ageism in our culture, would be called *gerontophobes*—our word.

Language is a boxing match in which you must spar daily, warding off negative suggestions that age is your worst enemy. Indeed, it is your best friend.

The aim of this book is to help you emphasize health and vigor, the aura of life and energy surrounding a person, not the person's age: not how old he is, but how vibrant he is. And begin to speak of age in positive terms, thus enhancing your ability to think positively about the inevitable process.

def•i•ni•tion

A **genarian** is anyone in their 60s, 70s, 80s, or 90s.

Sexagenarians are in their 60s; **septuagenarians** are in their 70s; **octogenarians** are in their 80s; **nonagenarians** are in their 90s; and **centenarians** are over 100.

Gerontophobia is an illness stemming from age anxiety and the fear of getting older.

The Least You Need to Know

♦ Age quotients are a better indicator than chronological age of our true age.

♦ Age, like time, is relative.

♦ Decrepitude isn't natural to aging.

♦ Advertising is awash with ageisms.

♦ The words you use affect your attitude toward aging.

Chapter 2

What Is "True Age"?

In This Chapter

- ◆ Discovering your true age
- ◆ Taking the quizzes
- ◆ Scoring your answers
- ◆ Examining your results

Discovering your true age is an illuminating process. It's also a lot of fun. The requirements to do so are simple. All you have to do is keep an open mind, be honest with yourself, answer as many questions as you can, and keep your calculator handy!

True Age Discoveries

We have been conditioned to view certain characteristics as youthful (enthusiasm, indecisiveness, adaptability, etc.) and others as old (rigidity, cynicism, obstinacy). We tend to be dismissive of older people. Discovering your true age will help you recognize that the many characteristics associated with various age groups have no "age" per se.

The general premise upon which the age quotient evaluations are based is that any behavior or activity leading to growth and expansion, humanism, enlightenment, and health is mature behavior. As such, they will give you an "older" age quotient. Behavior or activity that in any way blocks or constricts your evolution as a fulfilled human being is immature and will give you a "younger" AQ. These are not hard-and-fast rules; there are some exceptions, as you will see in the section on optimal age quotients later in this chapter.

Each chapter in Parts 2, 3, and 4 begins with a quiz that is designed to help you raise your "age consciousness." The main point of this book is that each of you possesses several ages at the same time, each age springing from a different aspect of your life. We call these aspects "age quotients," and there are 13 of them. Think of your chronological age as the pole star around which there are 13 directions. You can travel from one direction to another, or back to the pole star. It is the center, the stable point in the many journeys—or ages—of your life. The journeys reflect your true life experiences—your true age—but the pole star is always there.

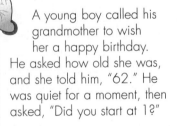

Wisdom of the Ages

A young boy called his grandmother to wish her a happy birthday. He asked how old she was, and she told him, "62." He was quiet for a moment, then asked, "Did you start at 1?"

When you complete all of the quizzes, you will have all your AQs, which is how we'll be referring to age quotients from here on. From these 13 AQs, you will be able to figure out your true age.

Those who insist on the absolute value of chronological age may sneer at the notion of a true age. But before you put this book aside, think of how you would complete the following sentence:

"A middle-aged person is too old to ..."

- ◆ Start a new career.
- ◆ Change his lifestyle.
- ◆ Have a baby.
- ◆ Go back to school.

- ◆ Take up rollerblading.

- ◆ Begin a love affair, especially with a younger person.

- ◆ Travel alone, especially if the person is a woman.

If you picked even one of these endings, you've been influenced by age stereotypes that have nothing whatsoever to do with your personal frames of reference. Stereotypes are barriers that keep us from the full realization of our potential.

In Parts 2, 3, and 4 we attempt to break through those barriers by exploring 13 age quotients.

The Quizzes

Each chapter begins with a brief quiz. Be as thoughtful and as thorough as you can with each. You may sometimes find a question that does not pertain to you and you cannot answer it. Don't worry about it. Scoring takes into account the number of questions you answer for each section. But the more questions you answer, the more the results will reflect who—and how old—you really are.

You will also find one chapter or another that does not pertain to you. If you are not in a romantic relationship, you will skip the significant other chapter (Chapter 11) and figure out your singleness AQ (Chapter 10) instead; and if you have a significant other or spouse, you will skip the singleness chapter.

You will notice that the answers have letters next to them, and that the letters are not sequential (A, B, C, etc.) but instead seem scattered (G, A, D, etc.). Some answers even have the same letter—there might be two "B"s or three "G"s. That's because in our scoring system (explained later in the chapter) each letter has a different value, and sometimes two different answers have the same value.

There is no right or wrong answer. Each quiz is meant to help you realize your true age on a sliding scale. Sometimes you'll want it to be "young"—and sometimes you'll want it to be older, meaning more mature!

Use the tabulation boxes that follow the quiz in each chapter. They do require a little simple math, so you might want to keep a calculator handy. When you've gotten through all 13 age quotients, you will be able to figure out your true age using the scoring box on the inside back cover of this book.

Optimize Your AQ

You might want to make copies of the quizzes and tabulation boxes so that others with whom you share this book can also take the quizzes. Photocopying the quizzes will also enable you to take them again yourself, which you may wish to do after finishing the book.

The quizzes are not scientific or clinical verifications of your various ages. Instead, they are guideposts to assist you in raising your age consciousness. They are designed to help you become aware of the various age barriers you may have built around yourself, mirroring the ageist attitudes so rife in this society.

Optimal AQs

Here is a summary of optimal age quotients for each of the age categories covered in this book:

- ◆ **Medical and physical fitness AQ:** Everyone wants to look and feel her healthiest. But the more years you have to indulge in the deleterious effects of "the good life," the more vulnerable the body is to deterioration. Ideally, the 20- to 35-year range is what to shoot for. But you really have to look at these AQs on a sliding scale, depending upon your chronological age, with a goal of at least 20 years younger.

- ◆ **Sexuality AQ:** Because most people need time and experience to fully explore their sexuality and to be comfortable and open in their sexual relations, you may want to work toward an optimal range of 30 to 45.

- ◆ **Brain fitness AQ:** Your brain isn't fully developed until you reach your mid-20s, so you don't want a brain true age younger than, say, 25.

- ◆ **Self-image, spirituality, and future AQs:** Because each of these AQs signals a combination of inner exploration, self-knowledge, interconnectedness, and planning, a very mature true age is desirable. If your true age is over 60, you're definitely going in the right direction; if it's 70 or 80, you are clearly at the top rung of Maslow's Hierarchy of Needs (see Chapter 8).

◆ **Significant other, family, and social AQs:** Aim for a true age over 40 with these "outer circle" AQs. That is indicative of mature, solid relationships that haven't gone stale.

◆ **Financial and community AQs:** Here, anything over an AQ of 40 certainly shows you've got your feet solidly on the ground; if it goes up to 50 or 60 or even higher, so much the better.

Scoring

Here's how to figure out your age quotients. With a calculator in hand and using the tabulation boxes that follow the quizzes in each chapter, follow these simple steps:

1. Write in the letter for each answer in the corresponding space. Then write in the value of points for each letter; the values are as follows:

    A = 5 B = 15 C = 25 D = 35 E = 45 H = 55 I = 65
    J = 75 K = 85

Here's an example:

	Medical True Age	
	Letter	Points
1.	B	15
2.	F	55
3.	D	35
4.	D	35
5.	C	25
6.	H	75
7.	C	25
8.	H	75
9.	F	55
10.		
11.		
Total		395
÷ #?s		9
AQ		43.8

Sample tabulation box.

2. Add up the points and write the total in the corresponding space.

3. Write in the number of answers you responded to in the corresponding space (the one that looks like this: ÷ #?s); then divide that number into the sum of points.

The result is your age quotient. Write it in the corresponding space, in the column provided in the chapter.

Your True Age

After you've gone through all the chapters and have taken all the quizzes pertinent to you, enter all of your AQs in the table on the inside back cover and calculate your very own age profile.

> **Wisdom of the Ages**
>
> Oh you're as old as you think you are, if you think at all …
>
> —TV's *The Smurfs*

As you take the quizzes, try to assess yourself as realistically as possible. There will be times when you must generalize, however. For example, your relationship with your children or your parents is probably different with each parent and each child; just use the broad strokes here. If you have trouble deciding on an answer, choose the one that applies *right now*. Or decide to make it pertain to one parent or one child. These quizzes can be taken again and again. Your immediate responses are what count. It's a way to find out about yourself, to open up, to get in touch, and to explore!

The Least You Need to Know

♦ Some of your age quotients will be much "older," and some much "younger," than your chronological age.

♦ Your true age profile distinguishes you from others.

♦ Your true age is formulated from all your age quotients and your chronological age.

♦ Taking the quizzes requires only candor and a calculator.

Part 2

Physical Age Quotients

The age quotients in this part of the book have to do with your physical well-being—your medical, physical fitness, brain fitness, and sexuality true ages. Most people's initial reaction is to want to see these age quotients be younger than their chronological age. After all, if you're 40, you don't want to have a physical fitness AQ of 60! But don't be too quick to make such assumptions. Do you really want the brain fitness AQ of an 18-year-old? After all, Einstein didn't develop his theory of relativity until he was in his mid 20s. And Shakespeare's most prolific productions began at age 26 and didn't end until he was 49! Insofar as one's sexual AQ, be honest: Was sex really more satisfying at 18 than at 35? Or was it simply more obsessive or frequent?

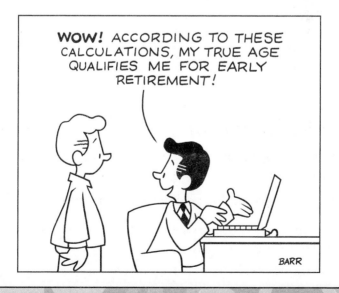

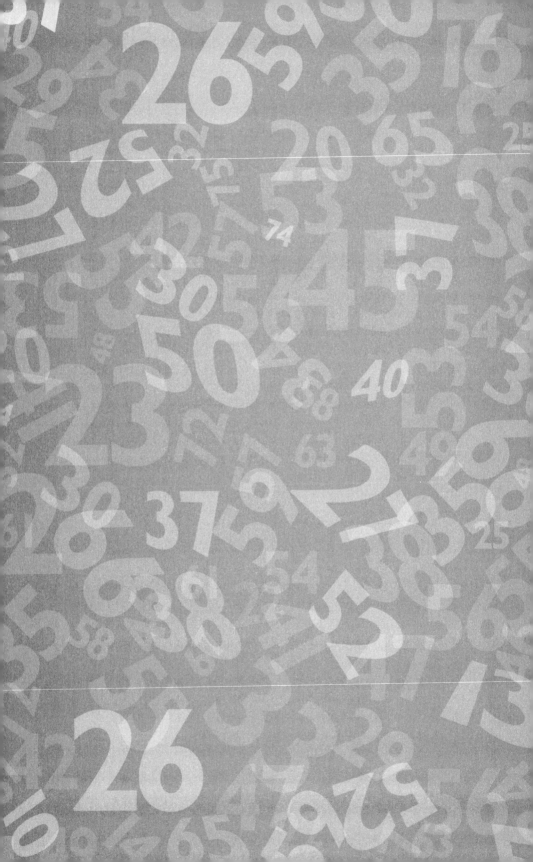

Chapter 3

Medical True Age

In This Chapter

- Optimizing your medical age quotient
- Dealing with disease
- Lowering blood pressure
- Controlling your body weight
- Learning to de-stress

You never really lose your youth. How can you? The experiences and lessons of youth belong to you. What you can and often do lose is vigor: well-toned muscles, a springy step, clear eyes, a glowing complexion. Although a certain degree of loss of vigor is inevitable as you get older, the good news is that the degree to which that happens is very much in your power to control.

Physical fitness, covered in the next chapter, deals with the results of healthful activities—what you should continue or start doing. Your medical AQ, the topic of this chapter, covers the results of bad habits and risky health indicators. (If you've already developed lots of good health habits, you'll whiz through this chapter.)

Your Medical True Age Quiz

1. How often do you have appropriate physical checkups?

   C. At regular intervals

   E. Occasionally, but not regularly

   G. Never or hardly ever

2. How many chronic conditions do you have (e.g., arthritis, thyroid disease, hypoglycemia, hypertension, etc.)?

   I. Two or three

   F. One

   J. Four or more

   B. None

3. Other than for normal childbirth, have you ever been hospitalized for illness?

   B. Never

   D. One or two times

   F. Three or four times

   H. Five or six times

   J. Seven or more times

4. How is your blood pressure?

   J. Very high

   G. On the high side

   D. Within the norm

   B. Optimal (120/80)

   C. On the low side

   F. Very low

5. Which of the following would you consider yourself?

    J. Obese (50 pounds or more overweight)

    G. 25 to 49 pounds overweight

    F. 5 to 24 pounds overweight

    B. Just right

    C. 5 to 19 pounds underweight

    G. 20 pounds or more underweight

6. Which best describes the way you usually feel?

    J. Very tense

    H. Fairly tense

    C. Fairly relaxed

    A. Very relaxed

    F. I go up and down all the time

7. What is the general state of your health?

    B. Excellent

    C. Very good

    D. Good

    E. Fair

    H. Below par

    J. Very poor

8. What are your smoking habits?

    A. Never smoked

    B. Quit at least five years ago

    C. Quit within the last two years

    J. Two to three packs or two to three cigars a day

    I. One pack or one cigar a day

    G. Less than one pack a day

    E. On rare occasions

9. How much liquor do you consume? (A drink equals one 12-oz. can of beer, one 4-oz. glass of wine, or one shot of hard liquor.)

    B. One drink on occasion

    C. Two to three drinks a week

    D. Four to six drinks a week

    G. Two to three drinks a day

    H. Four or more drinks a day

    A. Never drink

10. How often do you suffer from joint pain?

    J. Daily and throughout the day

    I. Daily but briefly

    H. Once or twice a week

    G. Once or twice a month

    E. A couple of attacks a year

    B. Rarely or never

Scoring

Here's how to score your quiz:

1. Write in the letter for each answer in the "Letter" column.

2. Using the Letter Values, find the value of points for each letter and write that number in the "Points" column.

3. Add up the points and write the total in the corresponding space.

4. Write in the *number of answers* you responded to for the section in the corresponding space (the one that looks like this: ÷ #?s) and divide that number into the sum of points.

The result is your medical true age!

Letter Values

A = 5 B = 15 C = 25 D = 35 E = 45 F = 55 G = 65 H = 75 I = 85 J = 95

Medical True Age		
	Letter	Points
1.		
2.		
3.		
4.		
5.		
6.		
7.		
8.		
9.		
10.		
Total		
÷ #?s		
AQ		

Interpreting Your Score

Where did you come out? If your medical AQ was at least 10 years younger than your chronological age, you can consider yourself in good health; if it was 20 or more years younger, you're batting a thousand! Of course, if you are in your 20s or 30s, that rule will not apply. But if you're like one 33-year-old single woman who took our online quiz and came up with of a medical AQ of 26, you're doing swell. Unlike the 21-year-old student who had a medical AQ of 41: smoking and 25 extra pounds of weight put him way behind the eight ball.

The next few pages will help you discover ways you can optimize your medical AQ by lowering it if you're older or equalizing it if you're younger.

Is Aging a Disease?

The state of your medical health is concerned with such big-ticket items as dietary habits, weight, alcohol consumption, smoking, and important measurements like blood pressure and cholesterol.

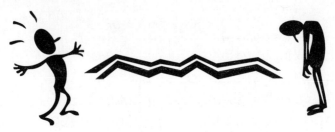

Continuum of optimal health to decrepitude.

At opposite ends of a long spectrum are optimal health and decrepitude. Many scientists and gerontologists question the assumption that aging leads to decrepitude. The growing field of anti-aging medicine is convinced that many people will live into their 100s in the very near future. But the main thrust of anti-aging isn't so much living longer as living *better.* As anti-aging expert Dr. Philip Lee Miller says, "Extending the prime of life is about growing older without aging."

Despite amazing advances in medicine, Americans are not a particularly healthy people. Compared with accidents, which are responsible for a little over 4 percent of all deaths, heart and related circulatory diseases cause more than 35 percent of all deaths; cancer causes more than 22 percent (according to the 2004 National Vital Statistics Report). So what can you do about it?

Lots. You may not be able to do anything to affect national statistics, but you can do a great deal to improve your medical AQ.

Your Own Drumbeat

One of the best clues there is to the health—and therefore the "age"—of your circulatory system is your blood pressure. What is blood pressure, anyway, and why is it so important? All the blood in your body, which is about 7 pints, passes into your heart and is pumped out again, making a complete circuit every 20 to 23 seconds (think Indy 500 sped up). Your blood pressure has two values: systolic and diastolic. Systolic reflects the high pressure, when your blood pumps out; diastolic reflects the low pressure, when it relaxes, allowing the blood to flow back in.

If you haven't had your blood pressure checked lately, do so, and have it checked regularly (many pharmacies offer it as a free service). Following is a chart showing blood pressure readings:

Blood Pressure Classification Chart (Adults)

Category	Systolic Pressure	Diastolic Pressure
Optimal	Less than 120	Less than 80
Normal	120–130	80–85
High-normal	130–140	85–90
Mild hypertension	140–160	90–100
Moderate hypertension	160–180	100–110
Severe hypertension	180 or more	110 or more

Ref: NIH Publication No. 98–4080, November 1997 (U.S.).

Hypertension is chronic high blood pressure. Your heart over-works when you have high blood pressure. Imagine trying to run a mile wearing a tight corset—your lungs would be at the bursting point. That's similar to what happens when your heart has to pump too hard.

Birthday Blahs

Shoot for the optimal blood pressure of 120/80. A reading over 140 systolic or 90 diastolic is high. See your primary care physician (PCP).

The greatest contributors to high blood pressure are not advanced age but obesity and high cholesterol. You can keep your blood pressure close to optimum in the following ways.

Eat a Heart-Healthy Diet

Eating a heart-healthy diet means limiting foods high in fats and cholesterol, like juicy steaks and scrambled eggs. Instead of slathering butter on your biscuit, use margarine or low-fat cottage cheese. In fact, forget the biscuit. Go for a whole-grain bran muffin instead.

When you cook, use olive oil. Avoid bacon and gravies. Use only low-fat or nonfat dairy products. Eat lots of raw fruits and vegetables. Get your protein from beans. Eat reasonable portions. Moderating ingestion promotes beneficial digestion. Drink water.

Get Regular Exercise

It doesn't matter if you walk, jog, or dance. Just get out there and do it! Thirty minutes a day would be perfect—even if it's done in small bites (a 15-minute walk and 15 minutes of bicycling). If you can't do it every day, set a schedule you can sustain, be it once or twice a week. The important thing is to begin—and stick with it. And drink water.

Birthday Blahs

Watch out for a distinct pain or cramping in your calf when you're out walking. If the pain goes away when you stop for a few minutes, then comes back when you continue, head to your doctor's office—this could be a symptom of peripheral arterial disease.

Okay, so it's snowing out. Change course! Climb the stairs in your apartment building. Do some rock-and-roll dancing. Just get your body moving, your heart beating, and your blood circulating.

Follow These Simple Rules

In addition to eating more healthfully and exercising regularly, you can ensure healthy blood pressure by sticking to the following guidelines:

♦ Know your blood pressure. Have it checked regularly.

♦ Avoid salty foods.

♦ If you're on blood pressure medicine, take it exactly as prescribed; never skip a day.

♦ Follow your doctor's advice about physical activity.

♦ Drink lots of water.

A Pound of Flesh

If you happen to be 20 pounds or more overweight and were offered a year of life for every 5 pounds you could shed, how much would you be willing to safely lose? Ten pounds would bring you two years; 20 pounds would bring you four! Body weight plays a highly significant role in the health and longevity of human beings. Other than our poor overfed pets, humans are the only mammals with obesity problems. To maintain a youthful medical AQ, make a tacit agreement with yourself to keep your weight down. (If it's already down, you can ignore this section.)

It isn't only the lowering of caloric intake that can lower your medical AQ: they must be the right calories. A 1,000-calorie-a-day diet of french fries and diet soda may reduce your weight, but it is not going to increase your life span.

Obesity is a highly significant factor in another all-too-common disease: adult-onset diabetes. In most instances, this occurs in people who are overfed, underactive, and overweight. And while significant improvement in any one or more of these areas may not eliminate the disease, it will at least hold it at bay.

High cholesterol levels cannot be overlooked, either, although they are not necessarily tied in to being overweight. There is "good" cholesterol, which is high-density lipoprotein (HDL), and "bad" cholesterol, which is low-density lipoprotein (LDL). You should be able to obtain a report of these levels from your primary care physician. (If you haven't been tested, please do so.)

Birthday Blahs

Reducing calories while still consuming foods high in fats and refined carbohydrates is dangerous to your health.

Understanding Cholesterol Levels

Element	Optimal	Borderline	High Risk
LDL cholesterol	<100	130–159	160
HDL cholesterol	60	35–45	<35
Triglycerides	<150	150–199	200
Total cholesterol	<200	200–239	240

Ref: National Heart, Lung, and Blood Institute.

You do not want to be in the borderline range, especially at the high end of it. Always shoot for the optimal range to help you gain a medical AQ you can gloat about.

Dealing with Stress

In today's climate of alarmist news, technological overload, crammed calendars, and daily deadlines, it's hard *not* to get stressed out. You may start the day feeling great, but by sundown your shoulders are up to your ears and the sudden honking of a horn may cause you to jump out of your seat. Tension is a killer. But there are ways to diffuse the stress pileup. Following the preceding dietary and exercise suggestions is a great beginning, but there are even more ways you can help yourself.

First, realize you can't avoid stress. The late Dr. Hans Selye, renowned stress expert, once observed that the complete absence of stress is death. Change brings about stress. Whether it's positive (marrying, a career change, moving to a new house) or negative (the death of a loved one, financial loss, natural disaster), it is still change. Change requires adaptability and coping powers. Selye's research made it very clear that the inability to cope with stress can literally destroy your organs. So how do you de-stress?

How Many Candles?

This web developer is a video-game junkie. He smokes, but not heavily, drinks a bit more than he should, has low blood pressure, and feels fairly tense much of the time (medical AQ 39). He skips meals, doesn't sleep well, and even though he's physically active several times a week, he's out of breath after one flight of stairs (physical fitness AQ 39). He's been faithful to the same woman for six years, but they each live in their own apartments. They have a great relationship, but are too dependent on one another (significant other AQ 34). He's very close with his family, who provided a warm and supportive upbringing (family AQ 46). While he enjoys going out with his friends, he doesn't find them entirely fulfilling. Shy in public, he likes spending evenings at his computer (social AQ 44). He reads a lot, does all kinds of puzzles, and really oxygenates his brain with daily exercise (brain AQ 19).

Well-educated with a decent job, this man's true age is 43. His chronological age: 21! If this young fellow would quit smoking and start eating a healthy diet, he could lower those AQs and attain a true age more reflective of his youth.

Lots of low-key activities are quite effective stress relievers, including ...

- A walk before dinner.

- Yoga stretches in the morning.

- A long, warm bath.

- A good book.

- Bird watching, even in the city (pigeons are very amusing creatures).

When you're stressed out, your adrenal glands jump into action, increasing your heart rate so that your blood supply is elevated. This is good when you need a spurt of energy. But if every day feels like an emergency, you're going to suffer adrenal exhaustion. Herbal remedies and supplements can help adrenaline stress, like chamomile tea or the hormone DHEA (always check with your doctor before starting on supplements). To begin with, just taking a moment to drink a glass of water and hydrate yourself can make a big difference in how you feel.

Here's a simple relaxation technique that you can do almost anywhere:

Take a deep breath. Sit back in your chair, lean your head back, and slowly breathe out. Close your eyes. Let your mind float. Allow a peaceful picture to enter your mind's eye—the ocean, a meadow, a sleeping baby, a litter of puppies. Hold that image for a moment or two while you breathe regularly. Now gently roll your head back and forth, relaxing your neck and shoulders. When you're ready, open your eyes.

This technique takes barely any time at all, yet it can slow your heart rate and give your body a little respite. It's amazing how positively your body—and your brain—responds to some form of relaxation exercise done two or three times a day.

Sometimes stress is so overwhelming that you can't de-stress without assistance. *Biofeedback* training, available at many physical therapy clinics and medical centers, uses the mind to control the body. It has been shown to be helpful in treating about 150 medical conditions. Or you could try transcendental meditation. If you're feeling too out of control, consider seeking out a good psychotherapist. The important thing is to find a way to de-stress: relaxation is a powerful healer.

def•i•ni•tion

Biofeedback is a method for learning to increase one's ability to control biological responses, such as blood pressure, muscle tension, and heart rate. Sophisticated instruments are often used to measure physiological responses and make them apparent to the patient, who then tries to alter and eventually control them without the aid of monitoring devices.

The Vise of Vice

The things people do to themselves! Popping pills, drinking, smoking: everyone knows they shouldn't, but that doesn't always stop them. You have the power to monitor yourself, but sometimes you need a little reminder.

Pill Mania

In trying to deal with stress, anxiety, weight gain, and insomnia, many people use pharmaceutical remedies. Once in a while may not be an issue. But if you find, on a daily basis, that you're popping amphetamines, barbiturates, and tranquilizers, not to mention over-the-counter drugs like antihistamines, sleeping pills, aspirin, and what have you, you might want to stop and think about it. These chemical catalysts can have an injurious effect on hormone production and blood pressure. All your good efforts of exercise and diet can go kaput!

Instead of sleeping pills, have a glass of warm milk, or hot water with lemon in it, or a cup of chamomile tea. Take a warm bath. Or try natural herbal supplements like valerian root and melatonin, though it's smart to check first with your doctor before self-medicating: even "natural" remedies have active ingredients that can be harmful.

Smoking Scandal

You know you shouldn't smoke. Smokers are at higher risk of heart attack, stroke, and various cancers of the lungs, throat, and mouth. Smoking is responsible for about one in five deaths in the United States.

Smokers like to point to the old codger of 87 who has been smoking four packs of Lucky's every day since he was knee-high to a tobacco leaf. But statistics prove this to be a rare exception. If you stop smoking, you can lower your lung's AQ by 10 to 15 years within two years!

 Optimize Your AQ

Within two years of quitting, you can completely reverse the damage done to your lungs by smoking.

Liquor Is Quicker

Unlike foods, which require time to digest, alcohol is metabolized extremely quickly by the body. Alcohol butts in line, absorbing and metabolizing before most other nutrients. About 20 percent is absorbed directly across the walls of an empty stomach and can reach the brain within one minute. Because it reduces the use of fats and carbohydrates, alcohol is highly toxic to the liver, where it leaves fatty deposits that can lead to cirrhosis, a chronic liver disease. Alcohol is also fattening!

Approximately 75,000 Americans die each year due to excessive alcohol use, making it the third leading lifestyle-related cause of death in the nation. If your consumption of alcoholic beverages interferes with physical and mental health and with family and social responsibilities, you are abusing it. Alcoholism is the most severe form of alcohol abuse. The NIAAA says a safe level of drinking for most adults is up to two drinks per day for men, and one drink per day for women or anyone whose reaction times have begun to slow. Of course, certain people, including women who are or trying to become pregnant, shouldn't drink at all. One drink equals one 12-ounce bottle of beer or wine cooler, one 5-ounce glass of wine, or 1.5 ounces of 80-proof distilled spirits.

If you're curious about your drinking habits, go to the American Council on Alcoholism and Treatment (www.aca-usa.org) and take a quick test.

The Change

Last but not least of the so-called "medical problems" affecting your medical AQ are the changes in male and female hormone levels that occur when you reach midlife. Estrogen, progesterone, and testosterone levels begin to taper off in both men and women.

How Many Candles?

This widow lives alone. She is a champion Scrabble player with a brain AQ of 44. Retired, she doesn't like to drive at night or on the freeway. She and her friends love dining at Chinese restaurants (friendship AQ 44). She flies to New York to see her son's family, and often visits her nearby daughter and grandson. Her health is good, though she has a little problem with numbness in her fingertips; her medical AQ is 39, and her physical fitness AQ is 49. She has a solid sense of herself (self-image AQ 88). Her true age is 72. Her chronological age: 94! Looks like this active genarian is doing everything right.

For women, the end of the reproductive cycle is menopause, when menstruation stops and they can no longer conceive. For most women this occurs between the ages of 45 and 52. Some of the symptoms experienced by many women include hot flashes, profuse perspiration, both of which may interfere with sleep, and a thinning of the vaginal wall, which may cause pain or discomfort during intercourse. Psychological fears of "losing one's womanhood," of "getting old," can promote symptoms of moodiness and depression. Your doctor can prescribe hormones and natural remedies to treat the physical symptoms. The psychological ones can be treated with a change in attitude.

In men, too, there are changes in hormone levels and "cycles" in what is now often termed andropause. Although more subtle than menopause, it may bring on symptoms ranging from dizziness to erectile dysfunction.

If you consider "the change" to be a harbinger of old age, self-doubt and worry may set in. Individuals may take to eating sweets or drinking as an escape from their fears. Finding the proper adjustments to hormone levels is one of the most powerful things you can do to slow biological aging. While there are many concerns about hormone replacement therapy (HRT), the risk is still considered slight by most professionals. Plus, sex hormones aren't the only ones that can help. Anti-aging specialist Dr. Philip Lee Miller calls these the "joie de vivre" hormones. There are many natural supplements that can help restore balance as well, such as black cohosh and soy. As always, a visit to your physician is advisable.

Wisdom of the Ages

He, who has health, has hope; and he who has hope has everything.
—Arabian Proverb

The beauty of achieving a healthy medical AQ 10 to 20 years younger than your chronological age is that you are in control! You can change your eating and drinking habits, lose or gain weight, quit smoking, and teach yourself de-stressing techniques. With a little effort, you can lower your medical AQ and feel a whole lot better in the process.

The Least You Need to Know

 ◆ Get an annual checkup.

 ◆ Make physical exercise a part of your regular routine.

 ◆ Eat well-balanced, healthy meals and watch your weight.

 ◆ Take a moment to defuse tension with quick, easy techniques.

 ◆ If you drink, limit your alcohol consumption; if you smoke, quit.

Chapter 4

Physical Fitness True Age

In This Chapter

- ◆ Optimizing your physical fitness age quotient
- ◆ Balancing nutrition
- ◆ Keeping your weight and body mass in check
- ◆ Testing your general fitness
- ◆ Building strength and endurance

Moderate exercise and balanced nutrition are the prime elements in achieving an optimum physical fitness AQ. With proper attention to physical fitness, there's no such thing as "middle age"—just another age, one still ripe with potential. In this chapter, you'll learn the simplest, most effective ways to optimize your physical fitness AQ.

Your Physical Fitness True Age Quiz

1. What is the condition of your skin?

    H. Very poor (for example: blotchy, scaly, acne)

    E. Mediocre (for example: no acne but dry and dull)

    C. Fairly good (for example: clear but not springy)

    B. Excellent (for example: springy and elastic; good moisture)

2. How are your sleeping habits?

    G. Suffer from chronic insomnia

    E. Sleep well, but less than seven hours

    F. Sleep long enough (seven to nine hours), but not well

    B. Sleep both well and long enough

3. When do you eat your meals?

    C. At regular hours

    F. Irregularly

    E. Often skip some meals

    G. Nibble throughout the day

4. Are your meals nutritionally well balanced?

    B. Most of the time

    F. Some of the time

    H. Not usually

    J. Never or hardly ever

5. For your age, what do you consider your physical strength?

    B. Well above average

    C. Somewhat above average

    D. Average

    G. Somewhat below average

    J. Well below average

6. How flexible are you physically? (For example, can you touch your toes, raise your arms above head, etc.?)

   B. Very flexible

   D. Fairly flexible

   G. Not very flexible

   I. Quite inflexible

7. Are you gasping and wheezing for breath after climbing ...

   I. Four to five steps?

   G. A flight of stairs?

   E. Two to three flights of stairs?

   C. Four to five flights of stairs?

   B. Six or more flights?

8. How often do you participate in active sports or exercise activities?

   B. On a daily basis

   C. Four to five times a week

   E. At least twice a week

   G. At least once a week

   H. Less than twice a month

   J. Never or hardly ever

9. Hold your stomach in a flexed, taut state, just as you might flex your biceps. How does it feel?

   B. Hard and muscular

   C. Firm and resilient

   D. Gives a little, but solid beneath

   H. Soft and mushy

   J. Too flaccid to hold in

10. What level of energy would you say you have now as compared with 10 years ago?

    A. 100 percent

    C. 80 percent

    E. 60 percent

    G. 40 percent

    I. 20 percent

    J. 10 percent

Scoring

Here's how to score your quiz:

1. Write in the letter for each answer in the "Letter" column.

2. Using the "Letter Values" list, find the value of points for each letter and write that number in the "Points" column.

3. Add up the points and write the total in the corresponding space.

4. Write in the *number of answers* you responded to for the section in the corresponding space (the one that looks like this: ÷ #?s) and divide that number into the sum of points.

The result is your physical fitness true age!

Letter Values

A = 5 B = 15 C = 25 D = 35 E = 45 F = 55 G = 65 H = 75 I = 85 J = 95

Physical Fitness True Age		
	Letter	Points
1.		
2.		
3.		
4.		
5.		
6.		
7.		
8.		
9.		
10.		
Total		
÷ #?s		
AQ		

Interpreting Your Score

Everyone wants to look and feel his or her healthiest. But the more years you indulge in the deleterious effects of "the good life," the more vulnerable the body is to deterioration. Ideally, the 20- to 35-year range is what to shoot for when it comes to your physical fitness AQ. But you really have to look at this AQ on a sliding scale, depending upon your chronological age, with a goal of at least 10 to 20 years younger.

For example, one man, age 43, had superior medical and physical fitness AQs—28 and 25 respectively. He neither smokes nor drinks, he exercises daily, has no chronic illnesses, eats and sleeps well, and is in excellent health. Yet a married woman of similar chronological age arrived at AQs within only one or two years of her chronological age; a lack of exercise and immoderate drinking kept her physical fitness AQ far from the ideal goal. At the other end of the spectrum, several genarians had physical fitness AQs down in the 30s!

Following is some sound advice on how to achieve a healthful physical fitness AQ.

Defining Physical Fitness

Just what is physical fitness, anyway? It is a state of optimal maintenance of strength and agility, as well as proper functioning of the internal organs. It is a state of vigor and zest. A body that's fit performs well,
resists disease, and stands up to stress. It means you can handle a physical emergency, like making it up the 12 flights of stairs at the office
when the elevator breaks down, walking home through heavy winds in
a snowstorm if the car won't start, being able to run or swim far enough
to save your own or another person's life. That's general physical fitness.

There are specific types of physical fitness:

◆ Muscle strength—Parents of babies and toddlers know how
important it is to have strong arms, legs, and backs. Firm, moderately developed muscles are essential, whether carrying groceries
or scrubbing out the bathtub.

◆ Endurance fitness—The ability to stay on task for however long it
takes to finish a project. Whether it's cleaning the house or completing a project report, endurance fitness is mandatory for making deadlines and achieving goals.

◆ Aerobic fitness—Aerobic means "to use oxygen"; aerobic fitness
maximizes the body's ability to take in and utilize oxygen. Not
only is this requisite to the jogger or public speaker, but it will
help keep your brain functioning optimally.

◆ Anaerobic fitness—Anaerobic exercises such as weight lifting and
isometrics help build muscle strength without using oxygen, the
way jogging or calisthenics do, and do so much more efficiently. It
comes in very handy if you're swimming underwater or singing an
aria, of course, but its uses are ubiquitous, allowing one to exert
strength even when at a standstill.

◆ Orthostatic fitness—The ability of the body to make sudden
changes in posture; any dancer or athlete would be lost without
it. But so would you. When you trip, it is orthostatic fitness that
helps you steady yourself without taking a bad tumble.

You might say relaxation fitness is necessary, too. The ability to voluntarily reduce the excess tension accumulated in the neuromuscular system makes it possible to cope with stress; what could be healthier than that!

Pessimists like to say you begin to die the day you are born. While it is true that some of your 60 trillion cells are dying all the time, some are being "born" all the time, too. Skin cells reproduce every 10 hours or so. Every 3 months your bloodstream is essentially replaced. Almost every cell in your body has renewed itself within 11 months, with the exception of bone cells—they take 2 years. This constant sloughing off and renewing of your cells gives you daily opportunities to maintain and promote good health, and to reverse poor health. Physiological aging can be slowed down and even reversed—and you're the one who can do it!

The Importance of Digestion

There are two basic tools for promoting physical fitness: what you do *with* your body, and what you put *into* your body. In order for food to do you any good at all, you must be equipped to digest it properly.

The digestive system is basically a plumbing system. It begins at the mouth, travels down the esophagus into the stomach, moves through the small intestines and the colon (the large intestine), and exits through the rectum, ending at the anus. It's a very long pipeline, utilizing many other organs along the way—liver, pancreas, kidneys, and bodily fluids such as saliva and gastric juices.

Aging in and of itself causes no significant impairment of the digestive system. What mucks it up is when it's mistreated. Then it springs forth with a barrage of ailments: heartburn (which has nothing to do with your heart), acid indigestion, ulcers,

Wisdom of the Ages

Take care of your body. It's the only place you have to live.

—Jim Rohn, motivational speaker

hemorrhoids, esophagitis (inflammation of the esophagus), irritable bowel syndrome, and lots more. The digestive system pays you back in kind for everything you do to it—energy and spunk in return for good nutrition and moderate consumption, sluggishness and misery for junk food and gorging.

Your body works very much like an internal combustion engine: ingested food is converted into energy by means of burning it as fuel. Each unit of energy that is burned is called a calorie. If you burn more calories than you ingest, you lose weight; if you burn fewer calories than you take in, you gain weight; if your caloric intake and expenditure is about the same, your weight will stay the same.

Food, Glorious Food

It's not only how much you eat, but *what* you eat that dictates the state of your general fitness. Food needs to supply you with calories, yes—but they must be the right calories. Your fuel formula needs vitamins, minerals, and enzymes, the basic building blocks of healthy living tissue. Much of this is stripped away by food manufacturers in an effort to provide convenience foods with long shelf life. But as the saying goes, "If mold won't grow on it, you won't grow on it," and if bugs can't survive in it, neither can you.

Optimize Your AQ

When you shop, avoid the center aisles and concentrate on the "fringe" foods, the stuff shelved along the perimeter of the market: produce, dairy, fish, and chicken: that's where you'll find your nutrition.

Eating habits have changed markedly over the decades. Prior to the turn of the twentieth century, the average per-person consumption of sugar was 5 pounds a year; now it's 142 pounds per year. (If you include high-fructose corn syrup, which flavors everything from frozen meals to fruity yogurt, it skyrockets to 203 pounds.) The U.S.D.A. reported that daily caloric intake between the years 1977 and 1996 had increased by an average of 143 calories for women and 268 for men. Oops, there's that extra 15 pounds. About two thirds of U.S. adults are overweight or obese. The proportion of U.S. children who are overweight has tripled since 1976, and now totals more than 9 million.

It's weird, but you can eat an abundance of food and still be undernourished. Good nutrition means balanced nutrition. Surveys show that 42 percent of Americans eat fewer than two servings of fruits and vegetables a day; five to nine servings are recommended. If you're like most

Americans, you're eating more food than you need, you're eating more nutritionally depleted foods than you used to, and you're eating more of the wrong foods than you should.

What is balanced nutrition? Every nationality, it seems, has its own guides and recommendations: Asian, Spanish, Arabic, Irish, the United States. Our favorite is the Mediterranean:

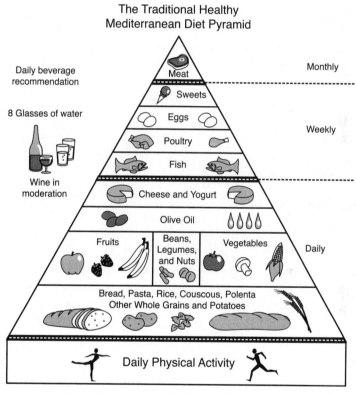

Mediterranean food pyramid guide.

Whichever country's food guidelines you choose, they all have certain basics in common:

♦ Eat plenty of fruits (2 to 4 servings), vegetables (3 to 5 servings), and whole grains (6 to 11 servings) every day.

♦ Reduce intake of *saturated fat*, *trans fat*, and cholesterol.

♦ Limit sweets and salt.

- If you drink alcoholic beverages, do so in moderation.

- Control portion sizes and total number of calories consumed.

- Drink plenty of water (8 glasses a day is recommended).

- Include physical activity in daily routines.

def•i•ni•tion

Saturated fat is a type of fat that's most often of animal origin. Trans fat is a type of unsaturated fat industrially created for the purpose of extending shelf life. Both types of fat promote bad cholesterol, as opposed to polyunsaturated fats like olive oil, which promotes good cholesterol.

People are frequently puzzled by what constitutes a serving size. How do you figure that one out? Depending on what's on the menu:

- **Breads, cereals, rice, and pasta:** One serving equals 1 slice of bread; $1/_2$ cup of cooked rice, pasta, or cereal; or 1 ounce (think of a shot glass full) of cereal.

- **Vegetables:** Servings are measured in cups rather than ounces. One serving equals $1/_2$ cup of raw or cooked vegetables or vegetable juice or 1 cup of leafy raw vegetables.

- **Fruits:** Like the vegetable group, cup size matters here, too. One serving equals 1 cup of fruit or 100 percent fruit juice, or $1/_2$ cup of dried fruit. But because fruits come in so many different shapes and sizes, it might help to think of the size of a tennis ball as one serving of whole fruit. For cut-up fruit, imagine a bowl of 5 to 7 avocado pits.

- **Milk, yogurt, and cheese:** One serving equals 1 cup of milk or yogurt, $1^1/_2$ to 2 ounces of cheese, and $1^1/_2$ cups of ice cream (do seek out low-fat options whenever possible).

- **Meat, poultry, fish, dry beans, eggs, and nuts:** Measured in ounce equivalents, one serving equals 1 ounce of cooked lean meat, poultry, or fish; $1/_4$ cup dried beans, after cooking; 1 egg; 1 tablespoon of peanut butter; or $1/_2$ ounce of nuts or seeds (think of that shot glass as half full now). So if you eat a piece of meat about the size of a deck of cards, that's 3 servings!

- **Oils:** Measure serving sizes in teaspoons.

Weight, Weight, Don't Tell Me

If you're at a good weight, you can skip this section. But if you need to take off a few pounds, give it a read.

It takes an exasperatingly small imbalance in the calorie intake/expenditure formula to make the needle on the scale go up. An extra half slice of toast at breakfast is 50 calories; that's 350 calories a week. In a year, it's 18,200 calories—equal to a $4^1/_2$-pound weight gain. If you decide to drive your new car to work instead of the brisk five-minute walk you used to enjoy, you will burn 18,200 fewer calories each year—another $4^1/_2$-pound weight gain.

The once-popular weight charts that showed averages for men and women of varying heights and frames, sometimes with 1-inch heels and clothing, other times barefoot and naked, are really a relic of the past. Today's physicians and fitness experts know that a more accurate key to a healthy weight is your body mass index (BMI), a much better indicator of health.

You could figure it out for yourself, but it's complicated. The easiest thing to do is go to the website of the National Heart, Lung, & Blood Institute at www.nhlbisupport.com/bmi, enter your height and weight, and you'll have it.

Here are some ways of burning off more calories during everyday routines:

◆ Use the stairs instead of the elevator.

◆ Park farther away from the store or office.

◆ If you use public transportation, get off one stop earlier.

◆ Instead of snacking, drink a glass of water.

◆ Speed-clean the house or speed-weed your garden.

◆ Dance when you listen to music.

Regulating caloric intake and expenditure is a matter of simple mathematics. It's one of the few aspects of modern life over which you have control. If you want to keep your physical fitness AQ at a vigorous low, then empower yourself with that control.

Checking What Kind of Shape You're In

There's a simple little test by which you may ascertain your general fitness. Take your pulse while you're at rest: the best time would be in the morning, before getting out of bed. If you've been sitting back watching TV for a while, that's a good time, too. You'll need a clock or a watch with a second hand. Gently place two fingers on the artery inside of your wrist, below your thumb. Don't use your thumb—your thumb has its own pulse. Count the beats for 20 seconds; then triple the result to get the number of beats per minute.

After this count, stand up quietly for just a moment or two, then take your pulse again. If it doesn't go up more than 15 counts, you're doing well. Now jog comfortably in place for about a minute. Then wait another minute, lie down, and immediately take your pulse again. If it's under 100, you're doing great!

Birthday Blahs

Ideal pulse rates for adult men are under 70, and for women, under 75.
If your resting pulse or heart rate is over 100, get thee to your primary care physician!

Normal ranges fall between 60 and 100 for adults, but these are not optimal. Well-conditioned athletes have heart rates of 40 to 60.

Keep Your Body Moving

Physical exercise helps keep your lungs, heart, and circulatory system in tune; it tones and develops your muscles, giving you a nicer shape; and it enhances your ability to relax fully, which includes improving the quality of your sleep. It lowers the incidence of cardiovascular disease, obesity, high blood pressure, and many other disorders.

Lean body mass diminishes because of inactivity, not aging. There are mountain-climbing *centenarians* in the Ecuadorean Andes who maintain their physical stature until death. Every day they climb and garden and carry heavy loads up and down the steep mountain slopes of their homeland.

Some people fear that physical exertion will increase their appetite. Nothing could be further from the truth. Cattle are penned because inactivity *increases* appetite, promoting rapid weight gain. The muscle tissue softens, body fat increases—great steak, lousy physical fitness. Exercise actually reduces appetite, particularly when it is done before meals. What's more, exercise increases circulation, and that promotes absorption of nutrients from food.

How Many Candles?

This big-city African American works as a clerk with a modest income. A moderate conservative, she is deeply religious, attends services regularly, and prays daily (spiritual AQ 83). She quit smoking a couple of years ago, enjoys two to three drinks every day, and is far too heavy for her height (medical AQ 41). She's not very flexible, despite her twice-weekly workouts, and feels her strength is below par. While she sleeps like a log, she doesn't eat regularly but nibbles throughout the day (physical fitness AQ 60). She's perfectly content with her single life (singleness AQ 32) and has a close and fulfilling circle of friends (social AQ 49). Not satisfied with her job, she's studying for a degree and wants to change her line of work (financial AQ 28).

Her true age is 59. Her chronological age: 29! Her true age has been boosted by very high medical and physical fitness ages—not a good thing. If they had been boosted as a result of very mature inner AQs, that would be different—and desirable. But as it is, this gal needs to adjust her eating habits, lose some weight, and moderate her drinking.

A minimum of 300 calories a day should be expended in some sort of conditioning program to get the optimum benefits. This chart shows caloric expenditure for different activities at different weights:

Calorie Burning Chart

Activity	Calories Burned in 10 min. at:			
	125 lbs	150 lbs	175 lbs	200 lbs
Aerobics (traditional at high intensity)	95	115	134	153
Cross-country skiing (2.5 mph)	26	80	93	106
Cross-country skiing (5–8 mph)	86	102	119	136

continues

continued

Activity	Calories Burned in 10 min. at:			
	125 lbs	**150 lbs**	**175 lbs**	**200 lbs**
Dancing (waltz, tango, etc.)	28	34	40	45
Gardening	41	49	57	65
Racquetball	75	90	105	120
Running (9 min./mile)	109	131	153	174
Shopping	35	42	49	56
Sitting (reading or watching TV)	10	12	14	16
Standing (light activity)	20	24	28	32
Swimming (vigorous)	95	113	133	152
Volleyball	28	34	40	45
Walking (15 min./mile)	44	52	61	70
Walking upstairs	150	175	202	229
Yoga (moderate Hatha)	26	28	33	38

Ref: Reebok Instructor News, Volume 4, Number 2, 1997 and The Fitness Jumpsite

Some experts say that the most beneficial cardiovascular and aerobic results come about when your heart rate is elevated to about 120 beats for at least 3 continuous minutes; quickly climbing three flights of stairs can get that job done. Other authorities, however, believe that a minimum of at least 15 minutes of activity, depending on what it is, is better. Our studies make us tend to agree with the latter.

If you're out of condition, your capacity for strenuous exercise has probably decreased, which means so has the safe range for maximum heart rate. How do you figure that out? A formula, of course! This one is simple:

Start with	220
Subtract	– <u>Your Age</u>
	Subtotal
For Safety	– <u>20</u>
Max. Heart Rate	Voilà!

You already know how to count your heartbeat from the discussion above. If you count for just six seconds and add a zero, you'll have your one-minute rate! Now, to be safe, do not exceed 20 beats per minute *less* than your maximum heart rate.

Some folks think that exercise is a great way to lose weight, but you'd have to jog a mile to lose just 1 ounce of body fat. Exercise promotes good health and a sense of well-being, but not necessarily weight reduction. Nonetheless, its benefits show up in the full-length mirror: muscle tissue, being denser than fatty tissue, takes up less space. And because exercise builds muscles, you can develop a trimmer silhouette without losing a single pound!

If you haven't participated in any regular program of physical conditioning and are now determined to do so, start slowly; long, brisk walks might be the best beginning. Let your physician know what you're planning, especially if you have any chronic health problems, and follow any recommendations he or she might offer. As the exemplary octogenarian Jack LaLanne says, "Do it—do it for life!"

 Optimize Your AQ

Treat your body like a child: guide it, feed it, exercise it, and care for it—then, like the bloom of youth, it will flourish.

By taking control of what you put into your body and what you do with your body, you can achieve a vigorous physical fitness AQ—one at least 10 to 20 years younger than your chronological years, if you're over 40, and at least 5 to 10 years younger if you're in your 20s or 30s.

The Least You Need to Know

◆ All aspects of physical fitness need maintenance.

◆ Balanced diet is essential for vigor.

◆ Body Mass Index is an important barometer of physical fitness.

◆ Resting and active heart rates are important indicators of physical fitness.

◆ For optimum physical fitness, exercise every day.

Chapter 5

Sexuality True Age

In This Chapter

- ◆ Optimizing your sexuality age quotient
- ◆ Becoming sexually mature
- ◆ Pleasuring yourself
- ◆ Experimenting sexually

Sex has come a long way since the Victorian notion of duty-bound babymaking. Society has moved from the tunnel vision of the first noted sexologist, Baron Richard von Krafft-Ebing, who believed sexual desire in "the old" to be a possible "precursor of senile dementia," to the panoramic scope of the Sex Information and Education Council of the United States (SIECUS), founded by Mary Calderone, who said: "Sex had to be brought out of the Victorian closet—freed from the guilt and fear, bigotry and misconceptions which shrouded it, if America was to recover from its deep-rooted sexual trouble." Thanks to SIECUS and other pioneers, it's no longer taboo to talk about sex—or enjoy it!

Your Sexuality True Age Quiz

As you complete the following quiz, keep in mind that "sexual activity" is a broad term, not confined to sexual intercourse. It includes masturbation, both by yourself or with a partner.

1. How often do you partake of sexual activities, alone or with a partner?

   B. Almost daily
   C. Two to three times a week
   D. Once a week
   F. One to two times a month
   H. Four to six times a year
   J. Never or hardly ever

2. In general, what is your response to these sexual activities?

   B. Enjoy it a lot
   C. Enjoy it somewhat
   H. Rarely enjoy it
   J. Never enjoy it
   E. Sometimes I enjoy it, sometimes I don't

3. If you have sexual relations with another person, how do you consider this person to be?

   F. Fair
   C. Wonderful
   A. Frustrating
   A. Exploitative
   C. Satisfying
   J. Miserable

4. How many people are you involved in a sexual relationship with?

    I.   No one

    D.   One person

    C.   Two different people

    B.   Three or four different people

    A.   Can't keep count

5. During sexual activities, do you experience orgasm?

    C.   Always, or almost always

    F.   Occasionally

    A.   Never or hardly ever

    B.   Yes, prematurely

    D.   Often; at least half of the time

6. What, if anything, leads up to sexual activities for you?

    C.   A romantic evening—dining, music, flowers

    B.   It's completely spontaneous; no lead-up at all

    E.   A regular time of the week

    G.   A lot of reminding from my partner

    D.   Sometimes it's C, sometimes it's B, sometimes it's a gentle suggestion from me or my partner

7. Do you engage in foreplay before sexual intercourse?

    C.   A lot

    D.   Somewhat

    H.   Rarely

    J.   Never

    E.   Sometimes I do, sometimes I don't

8. Do you enjoy kissing and hugging outside of sex?

    C.   A lot

    D.   Somewhat

    H.   Rarely

    J.   Never

    E.   Sometimes I do, sometimes I don't

9. What best describes your habits of affection?

   C. We kiss, hug, and hold hands a lot at home and in public

   D. We often hold hands in public, but never any other demonstration of affection

   B. We kiss and hug a lot, but only at home

   I. We have no physical contact except in bed

10. How do you feel after sexual activities?

    C. Relaxed and satisfied

    A. Guilty

    I. Resentful

    G. Frustrated

11. What is the status of frequency with your partner?

    H. My partner wants sex more than I do

    E. I want sex more than my partner does

    D. We both want sex with about the same frequency

12. Are you open to sexual experimentation?

    B. Eager for it

    C. Willing to try

    G. Too shy to try

    I. Wouldn't dream of it

Scoring

Here's how to score your quiz:

1. Write in the letter for each answer in the "Letter" column.

2. Using the "Letter Values" list, find the value of points for each letter and write that number in the "Points" column.

3. Add up the points and write the total in the corresponding space.

4. Write in the *number of answers* you responded to for the section in the corresponding space (the one that looks like this: ÷ #?s) and divide that number into the sum of points.

The result is your sexuality true age!

Letter Values
A = 5 B = 15 C = 25 D = 35 E = 45 F = 55 G = 65 H = 75 I = 85 J = 95

Sexuality True Age		
	Letter	Points
1.		
2.		
3.		
4.		
5.		
6.		
7.		
8.		
9.		
10.		
11.		
Total		
÷ #?s		
AQ		

Interpreting Your Score

Your sexuality AQ is based on how *you* feel about your sexual activities, not on what others think or what the often-exaggerated expectations of society are. If you believe sexual intercourse should occur only between married people in the "missionary" position, and you and your spouse have been happily married for years, enjoying intercourse on a mutually satisfying level, then you would still arrive at a mature sexuality AQ. If you believe sex is an art form that demands experimentation, then you, too, may have an optimal sexuality AQ. On a continuum from juvenile to very mature sexual relations, let's examine the sexuality AQ, with all its possibilities for growth and fulfillment.

Because most people need time and experience to fully explore their sexuality and to be comfortable and open in their sexual relations, you may want to work toward an optimal range of 30 to 45. What follows should improve your chances of doing so.

Sex Lore

There are major differences in sexual attitudes among varying age, economic, cultural, and political groups. Whether you're permissive or conservative in your sexual attitudes, it is your understanding of your own body, of what truly pleases you and your partner, that is a mark of sexual maturity, not chronological age or "experience." Frantic sex, inhibited sex, promiscuous sex, competitive sex, neurotic sex (like fetishism or sado-masochism)—these are immature manifestations of the sexual drive.

What dictates an optimal sexuality AQ? Here are some characteristics:

- ◆ Feel-good sex that doesn't compromise either person's health
- ◆ Knowing what gives you pleasure
- ◆ Uninhibited responses to receiving pleasure
- ◆ Knowing what gives your partner pleasure
- ◆ Joy in giving pleasure

What is an optimal sexuality AQ? That depends a great deal on your age and experience. You might think you want to have a sexuality AQ of 20, but if you're not 20, ask yourself this: was sex more rewarding at 20 than it was at 30 or 40? In the teens and 20s, while arousal may be swift and strong, inexperience and insecurity can truncate pleasures. For most people, sex becomes richer and more rewarding in their 30s and 40s, so a sexuality AQ in that range is quite desirable.

Full experience of one's sexuality and the intricacies of sharing with a partner can hardly come to fruition until one has been sexually active for at least 10 years. Some may brag that at the age of 48 they have a sexual AQ of 18—but it's unlikely their sex mates are bragging about them (unless they, too, are 18).

Although it is a debatable issue among sexologists, psychologists, and sociologists, we agree with those who include homosexuals in these definitions. Like heterosexuals, they may embrace a mature or an immature sexual lifestyle.

How Much Is Enough?

The frequency with which *coitus* takes place seems to be more socially conditioned than dictated by nature, varying widely from culture to culture. For example, in an island off Ireland, a researcher reports that frequency of sexual intercourse is best measured in terms of yearly incidence, whereas a Polynesian group in their 20s enjoy copulation 10 to 12 times a week; when they reach their late 40s, that figure falls to three or four times a week. Another researcher found that the African Bala have intercourse once or twice a day, right into their 60s!

There are dozens of studies surveying frequency of sex among men and women in different age groups, from teens on up to genarians. Frequencies vary so widely that they are meaningless in the face of your own sexuality AQ, which is about *you*, not about norms or averages. In other words, don't worry about it!

For most people, frequency of sexual activities begins to noticeably decline at around age 50, give or take a few years. Most women have approached

def•i•ni•tion

Coitus is sexual union between a male and a female involving insertion of the penis into the vagina.

Wisdom of the Ages

On his ninety-third birthday, fitness guru Jack LaLanne said, "I'm feeling great, and I have sex almost every day. Almost on Monday, almost on Tuesday, almost on Wednesday ...."

menopause by then, and most men are forced to recognize the onset of certain physical limitations. Even so, enjoyable sexual relations often continue into old age.

For post-menopausal women, the main problem they experience in sex is painful intercourse. This is due to a thinning of the vaginal wall and dryness. There are various ways of counteracting this condition:

♦ Take vitamin supplements that include A, B, and beta-carotene, as well as omega-3 essential fatty acids.

♦ Follow dietary regimes that include soy products (soy isoflavones help produce estrogen), and limit intake of alcohol, coffee, and tea, which tend to dehydrate.

♦ Drink water! Hydration keeps the cells plumped up.

♦ For hygiene, use pH-balanced soaps that do not include perfumes, antibiotics, or chemical deodorants.

♦ Topical estriol vaginal creams help boost the local estrogen and plump up the vaginal tissue.

♦ Use lubricants like Sylk or Astroglide. Even a dab of sweet almond oil or grapeseed oil can work.

♦ Balance the hormones by using estrogen replacement therapy and/or herbal remedies (check with your physician).

Birthday Blahs

Be sure to read the label of vaginal lubricants and buy only water-based vaginal lubricants. Avoid those that are petroleum-based (they can harbor bacteria and can cause damage to latex condoms) and those with methylparaben, a preservative that has been linked to cancer.

Some older men may experience difficulty in getting or maintaining an erection. Remedies like Viagra are available with a doctor's prescription.

With a willingness to deal with the particular challenges of sex for the older person, you can be successful in maintaining your sexual prowess right up through your elder years.

Masturbation

In her one-woman show, *Appearing Nightly*, Lily Tomlin jested that masturbation was something you do with the person you most love—

there are no problems of intimacy, and you don't have to get dressed up for it. Funny? Yes—and true. There is much to recommend the act of *autoeroticism.*

"Masturbation," wrote Thomas Szasz, is "the primary sexual activity of mankind. In the nineteenth century, it was a disease; in the twentieth, it's a cure."

It is popularly believed that most people stopped doing "it" when they were teenagers, if they did it at all. But the facts belie the myth.

> **def•i•ni•tion**
>
> **Autoeroticism** is self-satisfaction of sexual desire, usually by masturbation. It differs from masturbation in that the latter is excitation of one's own or another's genitals.

A major study done way back in 1975 showed that 82 percent of the women interviewed masturbate; out of the 1,844 women interviewed, only 56 did not reach orgasm. In psychotherapeutic terms, the discovery of their "inside" bodily selves correlates with women's discovery of their interior psychic selves. Another national study reported that 95 percent of men masturbate. Yet the practice is still widely condemned by several religious groups, including Mormons, Fundamentalists, and other Evangelical Christians; the Shi'a sect and some of the Sunni sects of Islam; and the Roman Catholic Church.

Old wives' tales of warts notwithstanding, masturbation is a common practice. Though frequency does seem to decrease with age, it is as beneficial in meeting the needs of the middle-aged and older person as those of the adolescent and young adult. The medical establishment today completely accepts masturbation as a healthy, natural adjunct of one's sexuality.

For the person without a sex partner, masturbation can provide a much-needed outlet for sexual energies. It can also enhance sexual activities between mates, serving as an excellent teacher as to what pleases. It can nurture in times of duress, anxiety, and sleeplessness. It is also a very special way to appreciate your own body, to enjoy it, explore it, and to let your body serve you, just as your mind and spirit do. When we refer to "sexual activities" in the questions at the beginning of this chapter, include masturbation in your consideration.

Other Aspects of Sex

Sex isn't all about intercourse, so even if penetration is problematic, there are many ways to enjoy your partner without it. A 65-year-old man, divorced and living with a younger woman, said, "Anybody who knows anything about sex knows there is so much more to it. Now, precisely because it takes me an hour to get a hard-on, I've had glorious sexual experiences during which I didn't even screw. Yet I felt loved and loving; I felt released. I felt all the other wonderful things that can happen. I am much richer sensually than I was as a young man, and I'm a much better lover."

A sprightly 72-year-old woman related another wonderful story of renewal. Her husband, after suffering a heart attack, developed an overly cautious approach to physical activity, including sex. For years, she tolerated his abstinence, respectful of his wishes and fearful of upsetting him. Then they decided to take a luxury cruise. Suddenly this busy woman found herself with a great deal of time to ruminate. She realized their relationship wasn't nearly as fun or rewarding since they had ceased their sex life. He was being too hesitant, she decided. She didn't want him to swing from the chandelier, just make gentle love. When she told him her feelings, he was genuinely surprised—and relieved. Talking about it released him from his fears. He practically threw her down on the bed and made love to her. Since then they've grown even closer—and have more fun.

How Many Candles?

This Swedish artist brought up two daughters single-handedly after her divorce. She rents a city apartment where she manages on a very modest income. Her work on huge sculptures is physically demanding, but she has kept herself fit (physical fitness AQ of 26; medical AQ of 38). She's close with her siblings, her daughters, and her new grandchild (family AQ 60). Living alone is acceptable to her (singleness AQ 38) but the good relationship she shares with a special friend is important (social AQ 46); her sexuality AQ is a mature 39. She keeps her mind sharp with daily reading, drawing, and three-times-a-week aerobics (brain AQ of 42). Her true age is 53. Her chronological age: 65. This woman seems to be doing everything right.

The smartest way to continue an active and satisfactory sex life as you grow older is to stop "groin-centered" thinking and reach out to more subtle and sensuous areas of sexual expression. Understanding the changes in sexuality as the years advance, not only in oneself but in the opposite sex as well, is key to maintaining a rewarding sex life.

"The basic human need for affectionate physical contact, which is apparent even in newborn infants, persists through life," writes John W. Rowe and Robert L. Kahn in *Successful Aging*. "The voltage is never too low for that," they continue. "In fact, it may help keep the lights on."

Before Foreplay

Most people are aware of the need for some sexual foreplay before intercourse takes place. Partners often start by holding one another and kissing. A woman's breasts may be caressed, or a man's penis stroked. They might have oral sex. But how much thought goes into what happens *before* foreplay?

Setting the stage for sexual adventure can be just as enjoyable and rewarding as planning the particulars of your annual vacation. A romantic dinner for two, a hint of perfume, music, slow dancing, rose petals on the pillow ....

Simply expressing your desires can be a turn-on. But many find it hard to talk about sex before, during, and after lovemaking. This reticence can lead to sexual frustration, dissatisfaction, and, all too often, resentment toward your partner.

Sex therapist Jackie Schwartz suggests removing the goal of intercourse as a major step in reviving a troubled sex life. The Los Angeles therapist persuades her clients to create a situation in which they can discover what gives them pleasure in a nonthreatening, nonsexual setting. A foot massage is one of the more popular methods she uses. Techniques such as this can help break old patterns, and put the zest back in your sex life.

Wisdom of the Ages

My husband walks in the door one night, he says to me, "Roseanne, don't you think it's time we sat down and had a serious talk about our sex life?" I say to him, "You want me to turn off *Wheel of Fortune* for that?"

—Roseanne Barr

Be adventurous, be daring, be willing to infuse your sex life with some variety, some eroticism, some laughter. Use various states of dress and undress, be vampy or look innocent, and have fun titillating your partner. Introduce a new toy into the act. Write a welcome-home greeting in edible body paint across your breasts or chest. Talk dirty. Sex toys such as vibrators, French ticklers, and flavored body creams can lend a playful air to sexual activities, diffusing the tensions of the day and adding to your pleasure. Try different positions. If you need some ideas, there are plenty of illustrated books to guide you—and to turn you on! Watch sex DVDs. Make a game of it: see who can wait the longest before having an orgasm, or see who can have one first!

One couple reported taking particular joy in locking the bathroom door at large parties and "having a quickie" while the guests caroused outside. Silly? Why not? Why shouldn't sex be silly and fun and light-hearted, as well as spiritual and deep? Why can't it be different things at different times? There's no real risk involved—you can always laugh it off if things don't work out, and try again another time. There is no right or wrong between consenting partners, as long as no harm is done to either.

To enjoy sex to the fullest, you must be in good physical condition. Sick bodies are not sexual bodies. Surely you've noticed that when you become ill, you lose your appetite not only for food, but also for sex. Here's an exercise that can help elevate your sexual pleasure.

The muscle that controls the genitals—the "sex muscle," if you will—can be strengthened and brought under control through isometric exercises. The next time you urinate, try to stop the flow midstream; hold it a moment, then release, and then stop it again. The muscle you are using is the "sex muscle." Once you've identified it, you can flex and release it at will while sitting at your desk or watching television. No one will know. Gaining control of this muscle can enhance enjoyment of sexual intercourse.

Exercises that keep the legs and torso strong and limber will enhance sexual capability. Even facial yoga exercises that strengthen lips and tongue can increase the pleasures of oral sex.

The road to a fulfilling and mature sex life is really the road of sensuality. Fully using all your senses prepares the body for enjoyable sex, just as exercising the mind prepares you for fulfilling your intellect.

The most workable key to a healthy sex life is taking a genuine interest in your partner and being completely honest with one another, both showing your strengths and revealing your weaknesses. When you're open and honest, affection will flow spontaneously and readily. With these kinds of approaches, you will no doubt find yourself achieving a mature sexuality AQ, one in accord with your chronological age or very likely "older."

The Least You Need to Know

 ◆ Groin-centered sex curtails full enjoyment of sexuality.

 ◆ Experimentation and playfulness enhances sexual relations.

 ◆ Masturbation is a healthy sexual outlet.

 ◆ Dealing practically and sensibly with menopause and andropause helps diminish their symptoms.

 ◆ Frequency of intercourse has little bearing on sexual satisfaction.

Chapter 6

Brain Fitness True Age

In This Chapter

- ◆ Optimizing your brain fitness age quotient
- ◆ Understanding how the brain works
- ◆ Finding out about memory
- ◆ Taking care of your brain
- ◆ Uncovering the heart-brain relationship

If you want to keep your brain fit, it's a good idea to first discover how the darn thing works! First, imagine the number of leaves on the deciduous trees in Yellowstone National Park (which covers 2,219,789 acres). Got the picture? Now you have an idea of the 100 billion nerve cells in your brain. Each of those cells is connected to around 10,000 others. So now try to imagine the number of pine needles on all the pine trees.

Just as all those leaves and all those pine needles and all those trees need specific conditions to stay shiny and healthy, your brain cells need specific conditions for high functionality. As you'll see, there are many things you can do to keep your brain working at its optimum best.

Your Brain Fitness True Age Quiz

1. How often do you read one book, or the daily paper, or four magazines (cover to cover, whether online or print media), or an equivalent combination?

   B. Once a week

   C. Twice a month

   E. Once a month

   G. Five or six times a year

   A. Daily

   I. Rarely or never

2. How often do you play word games (crosswords, Scrabble, etc.)?

   B. Daily

   C. Two to three times a week

   E. Once a week

   G. Occasionally

   I. Rarely or never

3. How often do you either play games of logic (Sudoku, bridge, jigsaw puzzles, Free Cell, etc.) or deal with spatial/logistical problems in your daily life?

   B. Daily

   C. Two to three times a week

   E. Once a week

   G. Occasionally

   I. Rarely or never

4. How often do you engage in hand-eye coordination activities (knitting, drawing, bowling, applying make-up, tennis, etc.)?

   B. Daily

   C. Two to three times a week

   E. Once a week

   G. Occasionally

   I. Rarely or never

5. How often do you engage in aerobic activities (walking, bicycling, singles tennis, calisthenics, etc.)?

    B. Daily

    C. Four to five times a week

    E. Two to three times a week

    G. Once a week

    H. Occasionally

    I. Rarely or never

6. How often do you listen to music, play music, or sing?

    B. Daily

    F. Two to three times a week

    C. Once a week

    D. Rarely or never

7. How often are you analytical, trying to understand your own or others' motives or state of mind?

    B. Always

    F. Often

    D. Occasionally

    E. Once in a blue moon

    C. Never

8. How often do you write or record in a journal or blog?

    B. Every day

    C. Two to three times a week

    D. Once a week

    E. Occasionally

    F. Once in a blue moon

    G. Never

9. How often do you continue your education by attending classes, workshops, lectures, or seminars?

   C. Once or twice a week

   D. Once or twice a month

   E. Six to eight times a year

   G. Two to four times a year

   J. Rarely or never

10. How has your memory changed over the years?

    B. Vastly improved

    C. Improved somewhat

    D. Remained much the same

    G. Deteriorated somewhat

    J. Deteriorated badly

11. How often do you have active contact with nature (gardening, bird watching, hiking, kayaking, etc.)?

    F. Daily

    D. Two to three times a week

    G. Once a week

    I. Once or twice a month

    J. Rarely or never

Scoring

Here's how to score your quiz:

1. Write in the letter for each answer in the "Letter" column.

2. Using the "Letter Values" list, find the value of points for each letter and write that number in the "Points" column.

3. Add up the points and write the total in the corresponding space.

4. Write in the *number of answers* you responded to for the section in the corresponding space and divide that number into the sum of points.

The result is your brain fitness true age!

Letter Values
A = 5 B = 15 C = 25 D = 35 E = 45 F = 55 G = 65 H = 75 I = 85 J = 95

Brain Fitness True Age		
	Letter	**Points**
1.		
2.		
3.		
4.		
5.		
6.		
7.		
8.		
9.		
10.		
11.		
Total		
÷ #?s		
AQ		

Interpreting Your Score

What's a good AQ for the brain? Well, you wouldn't want it too young because brains aren't fully developed until you're about 30. Lots of brainy folks do their best work at 50! So you certainly wouldn't want an AQ lower than 25. It is also known that, typically, brain function begins to deteriorate as you age. But you can slow that process down. If you're over 30, aim for a range between 30 and 45; if you're under 30, the lowest you'd want to go is 25. But there's no reason whatsoever you can't hit 45. If you'd like to optimize your brain fitness AQ, read on.

Brain Controls

Your brain is like the engine of a car. As the driver, you may think you're in complete control, but are you consciously circulating fluids, shuttling pistons, burning fuel? Nope. Same with your brain. It automatically controls your breathing, circulation, heartbeat, and burning of calories: you don't have anything to say about it. But there's a lot you can do to optimize those involuntary functions as well as the ones you can control.

The brain performs an incredible number of tasks, including the following:

◆ Controls body temperature, blood pressure, heart rate, and breathing.

◆ Processes a flood of information about the world around you from your five senses: sight, sound, smell, taste, touch.

◆ Directs physical motion: walking, talking, standing, sitting, sleeping.

◆ Thinks, dreams, reasons, imagines, and experiences emotions.

All of these tasks are coordinated, controlled, and regulated by an organ that is about the size of a small head of cauliflower.

The basic number of neurons in the brain is pretty well fixed by about age 20, and the slight loss people suffer as they age is negligible. It's not so much the *number* of neurons as the *health* of neurons that affects memory and reaction time. What's a major factor in keeping brain cells healthy? Oxygen!

Brain Responses

It's the brain's sensitivity to oxygen (or the lack of it) that gives you a hangover the morning after you've "tied one on" the night before. Like all the cells in the body, your brain receives oxygen via the red corpuscles in the blood. But before the blood can rush that fresh supply up there, the body's detoxifying organs—the kidneys and liver—have to clean things up. The keys to reversing this trend are:

- Oxygenation

- Brain energy

- Healthier neuronal membranes

- Protection of the brain

Reduction in oxygen to the brain can be caused by lots of things. But the most widespread and deadly is *arteriolosclerosis*, commonly called hardening of the arteries. In this condition, fatty deposits build up in the inner walls of the blood vessels, constricting the natural flow of blood to the brain (and elsewhere), which reduces the oxygen supply. What causes arteriolosclerosis? Many things, but prominent among them are inadequate diet and lack of exercise, both of which you have complete control over!

Science has shown there is a definite slowing of the conduction of nerve impulses in the elderly (i.e., slower reflexes). It is also not atypical that as people age, the neurons shrink and stiffen, chemical messengers decrease, and some vital connections are lost. Now this is a *very* gradual process that begins some time after age 30 and continues on until one expires. But it can be slowed even more, perhaps completely eliminated, if you take action.

def•i•ni•tion

Arteriolosclerosis is a chronic disease in which thickening, hardening, and loss of elasticity of the arterial walls result in impaired blood circulation.

 Optimize Your AQ

Physical exercise alone can reduce the probability of heart disease by about 30 percent.

Because the ability to respond quickly is essential to everyone, whether working at a desk, piloting a plane, or cooking a delicate omelet, learning how to rev up the brain is a worthwhile pursuit. A little more understanding of how our brains operate will be helpful in taking up the reins of that pursuit.

Understanding Memory

The brain is like a personal filing system, and it stores memories in three unique ways:

- ◆ Short-term memory
- ◆ Long-term memory
- ◆ Working memory

Understanding how these different kinds of memory work will help you see how important the brain exercises are that follow.

The dictionary defines memory as "the mental faculty of retaining and recalling past experience." The question is, when in the past? Five minutes ago? Five years ago? Fifty years ago? Most things are stored in your brain for only a short time—the names of people you meet at a party, for example. Unless you make special note of them or have contact again soon, you usually forget them. This is short-term memory.

Information can pass into your long-term memory, where it may stay for days, weeks, or even your whole life—like doing math, memorizing state capitals, the name of your first dog, and all the stuff you learned as a kid. Long-term memory is your personal history. There are different sorts of long-term memories—events, information, and how to do things, like brush your teeth.

Memories of things that have happened to you help you deal with the present and plan for the future. Your personal history, for instance, may forewarn you not to trust one person, and encourage you to befriend another.

Whether you "remember" something or not, everything you have learned and experienced is there—somewhere—in the databank of your mind.

How Many Candles?

A perennial student who also teaches computer skills, this woman is in good physical condition (physical fitness AQ 24), despite having been hospitalized several times. Even though she feels her memory has deteriorated, she keeps her brain fit (brain AQ 37) with daily aerobics, lots of reading, as well as spatial/logistic challenges, being quite analytical, and writing in her journal several times a week. She's not entirely satisfied with her work (financial AQ 39), but she does see room for advancement. However, she'd like to retire as soon as possible, though she has no idea what she'll do at that time. She has a whopping high future AQ of 76; she faces the future eagerly, welcomes new challenges, constantly seeks new horizons, and feels the pace of things are a bit slow for her. Her true age is 47. Her chronological age: 41! It may seem counter-intuitive that her true age is higher than her chronological age, but when one's level of maturity with the inner AQs (self-image, spiritual, and future) is very high, the result will boost the true age up, as you will see in Part 3. Aside from this woman's personal issues with her work, she is doing well on all counts.

Working memory is what you use when you're talking, washing dishes, or tying your shoelaces. It's what helps you drive a car without running off the road or hitting the gas pedal when you mean to hit the brakes. Your ability to instantly retrieve many different bits of information enables you to execute many functions automatically, without much forethought. Many researchers think that working memory is the key to human intelligence; it enables us to solve problems and plan ahead.

Wisdom of the Ages

First you forget names, then you forget faces. Next you forget to pull your zipper up, and finally you forget to pull it down.

—George Burns

Brain Aerobics

How many times, when you or someone you know forgets something, do you utter or hear the words, "I must be getting senile"? Much of the time forgetfulness is caused simply by a lack of oxygen to the brain, not senility. By increasing oxygen to the brain, you can reduce or even eliminate forgetfulness. There are many systems of exercise that will accomplish this task, but one that is significantly geared toward it is yoga.

In yoga, the practice of breathing, called *pranayama*, is considered to be the "life force." Even to Western thinking, there's nothing outlandish about that: bodies need to breathe to survive. Yoga practitioners believe that controlling your breathing is key to controlling your life.

Because deep breathing directly enhances the functionality of the brain, and the brain controls the body, yoga's ancient principles are very much in accord with several recent scientific discoveries. For example, lowered oxygen intake can lead to a slowing of protein synthesis, and that may be a factor in the lowered ability to learn and memory loss among some elderly. It has been shown that the breathing of pure oxygen can improve various mental processes; even the ability of the eye to adapt to darkness is improved by taking in pure oxygen.

How Many Candles?

A grandfather of five, this city-bred man now lives in a mobile home in a small town. His relationship with his wife has gotten better and better with the passage of years (significant other AQ 36). His medical AQ (35) would be better if his blood pressure weren't so high. Having worked for years as a mime, he is physically fit (physical fitness AQ 24). He does aerobics regularly, practices tai chi, enjoys puzzles and word games regularly, and engages in educational activities a couple of times a week; his brain AQ is 27. With a community AQ of 60, this fellow avidly follows politics and does volunteer work a couple of times a month. His true age is 62. His chronological age: 73! It's good that his marriage has improved, but an AQ of 36 is still a bit on the low side for such a long-term relationship. However, when it comes to the brain, he's doing everything right.

Developing lung capacity and practicing deep breathing can stave off many brain and memory dysfunctions brought about by low oxygen intake. The full use of your lungs will help optimize your brain fitness AQ. Here are some brain aerobics to help keep your noodle in tip-top condition:

◆ Stop what you're doing right now and take in a deep breath. Feel your shoulders and chest rise; when it feels like you've breathed in fully, take in a little more air. Now let it all out in a controlled flow. When you feel you've completely expired the intake, breathe out a little more. Repeat twice more. Do this two or three times a day.

- Lie down on your back near a wall or a chair. Put your feet up on the chair, keeping the knees relaxed and bent. If you can, put a pillow under your back, so your head is lower than your torso. Just stay there two or three minutes.

- Do an aerobic exercise for 15 minutes (jog, dance) or walk quickly up and down stairs for 3 minutes straight.

Body movement can also improve brain function. There is an organization, BrainGym.org, that uses the science of movement to enhance learning. Located in Ventura, California, they work with children, adults, and seniors, and claim their techniques help students to "learn *anything* faster and more easily, perform better at sports, be more focused and organized" and "reach new levels of excellence." This all emphasizes our point: movement and oxygenation to the brain is what you need.

Another movement exercise is the "cross-crawl," an excellent method for activating full mind-body function, especially for those with dyslexia, stroke, or other debilitating diseases. If you have been seated at the computer for hours, or even in an easy chair, your thinking may become sluggish, you may move awkwardly when you stand, and your energy may feel low. The cross-crawl changes that energy and enlivens you. Here's how:

Very simply, and as slowly as you can, stand in place, lifting the right leg and touching the knee with your left elbow. Back to standing, lift your left leg and touch it with your right elbow—slowly. If you can't quite touch elbow to knee, use your forearm. Do 10 to 20 repeats. When done on a regular basis (preferably daily), more nerve networks form and more connections are made in the corpus callosum, thus making communication between the two hemispheres faster and more integrated for high-level reasoning.

Brain Anaerobics

Getting oxygen up to your noggin is essential for good brain function, but how do you also keep it sharp? Your neurons need to be exercised in all parts of the brain. Brain anaerobics are the way to do it: word games (crossword puzzles, Scrabble), logic games (Suduko, bridge, jigsaw puzzles), and memorization (a poem, a witticism, a song) are all great exercise for the brain.

Enriching your immediate environment is another pathway toward keeping your brain fit. Experiments have found that laboratory rats placed with a large number of other rats in an enriched setting—a large cage equipped with ladders, mazes, tunnels, etc.—develop a thicker cerebral cortex than rats housed three to a plain cage. Putting time and effort into beautifying your environment actually increases your intelligence. What a deal!

Wisdom of the Ages

How old would you be if you didn't know how old you was?

—Satchel Paige

Get out in the fresh air, too. Breathe in nature. Scientists suspect that green space has a restorative effect on your voluntary attention, which means the ability to stay focused and ignore distractions, concentrating on the task at hand. Many experts believe that parks and gardens are essential to human social and psychological well-being. The time taken for that morning walk in the park will more than make up for itself with your increased ability to focus when you get back to work!

Optimize Your AQ

The brain fitness program comes from Posit Science in California. It's an expensive program (nearly $400) and requires effort, but it is effective. If you're interested, you can go to their website: www.positscience.com.

A new study suggests that one hour a day of intensive brain exercise can improve thinking and memory. Dr. Elizabeth Zelinski from the University of Southern California led a study of more than 400 people 65 to 93. Those who completed 40 hours of brain fitness training performed significantly better on memory tests than a comparison group who spent 40 hours watching educational lectures. People used their program for 1 hour a day, 5 days a week, for 8 to 10 weeks.

The Heart-Brain Connection

Oddly enough, another essential component of keeping your brain fit seems to have a lot to do with your heart. Researchers have recently discovered that the heart has its very own nervous system, with its very own neurons—about 40,000 of them—which participate in ongoing two-way communications with the brain.

The heart generates an electromagnetic field, just like the earth does. In fact, the heart generates 2.5 watts of energy: enough to keep a night-light going! While scientists don't completely understand this phenomenon, when you feel someone's vibes, you're probably picking up on this subtle heart energy. Perhaps people with "big" hearts are those who put out the most wattage—the true leaders.

Our sister, Susan Partnow, who teaches workshops in compassionate listening, says of this electromagnetic field, "It is our own personal weather system—together, collectively we create an ecology of emotion: we can contribute sunshine (love) or turbulence and dark clouds (fear, anger etc.)." Research shows it is actually contagious, she says, via *entrainment*, a law of physics.

def•i•ni•tion

Entrainment refers to how cycles tend to attune to one another: women living together end up with the same menstrual cycle; pendulums on grandfather clocks in the same room will, after a day, all be going in the same direction; heart cells from different organisms placed together in a Petri dish will begin to pulsate in concert. The stronger the field being put out (intense anger or deep love), the stronger the pull to others to get them into the same field.

This research confirms what poets have been saying for ages: a lot of emotion really does begin in the heart, not the brain. What's more, CAT scans show that heart activity generated by feelings of altruism and compassion actually have greater health-promoting effects on the immune system and the *autonomic nervous system* than any other emotional state—even inner peace.

So what does this have to do with brain fitness? Since there's a brain in your heart, and since positive emotions emanating from your heart sends positive messages to your brain, which then sends positive messages to your organs and

def•i•ni•tion

The **autonomic nervous system** is the part of the nervous system that regulates involuntary action, as of the intestines, heart, and glands.

glands, helping to keep you healthy and clear-headed, working at being positive is good for your brain. In other words, a loving heart is smart!

Once again, you are in charge. By simply practicing some of the exercises suggested, you can achieve a brain fitness AQ within the ideal range of 30 to 45 if you're over 30, and 25 to 45 if you're under 30.

The Least You Need to Know

◆ Your brain is the control engine of your body.

◆ Oxygen is the brain's fuel.

◆ There are three kinds of memory: short-term, long-term, and working memory.

◆ You can exercise your brain to improve functionality and optimize your AQ.

◆ Positive emotions are good for the brain.

Part 3

Your Inner Workings

It's time to turn inward, to find out what's going on inside that head of yours: your self-image, your spiritual life, your attitude, and preparation for the future. With these AQs, the older, the better. Mature AQs signify one who has done a lot of psychic homework and who possesses some hard-earned wisdom.

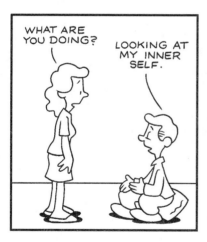
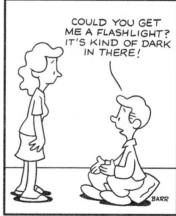

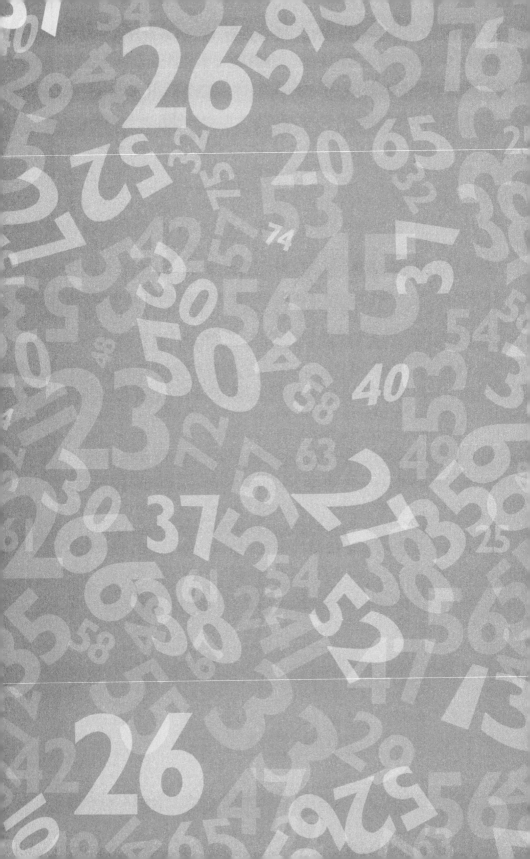

Chapter 7

Self-Image True Age

In This Chapter

- Optimizing your self-image true age
- Discovering how others see you
- Developing a positive attitude
- Learning how to accept yourself
- Dealing with loss gracefully

Bertolt Brecht, the masterful German playwright, once said, "I love those who change in order to stay themselves." But in order to stay yourself, you need to know who and what you are. This chapter delves into the elements that comprise a mature self-image AQ.

Your Self-Image True Age Quiz

1. How would you describe your age group?

   B. Just a kid

   H. A senior

   D. A mature adult

   F. Middle-aged

   C. A young adult

   E. One of the old folks

   J. An elder

2. In the past 10 years, how do you see yourself as having aged?

   G. Rapidly

   H. Slowly

   I. Steadily

   A. Not at all

3. How much does your age influence your interests and behavior?

   E. A great deal

   F. A fair amount

   H. A little bit

   B. Not at all

4. Without regard to cost or criticism, which of the following would be the first thing you'd do to look younger?

   I. Diet and exercise

   F. Dye hair and/or change wardrobe

   D. Cosmetic surgery or hair transplants

   H. Quit smoking and/or drinking

   J. Nothing; it's of little concern to me

5. How close does your physical image of yourself match what you see when you look in a mirror?

    I.   Just what I expected

    G.   Looks worse than I expected

    F.   Doesn't look as bad as I expected

    F.   Looks better than I expected

6. How content in your life are you now, compared with your younger years?

    J.   Much more content

    H.   Somewhat more content

    F.   About the same

    D.   Somewhat less content

    B.   Much less content

7. How do you rate this time of your life?

    J.   The best time

    B.   The worst time

    E.   No better or worse than any other

    H.   Getting better all the time

    D.   In a transitional time of life

8. How do you consider the middle years to be?

    J.   A time of growth and new experience

    B.   A time of despair and conflict

    C.   A static, nonproductive time

    E.   A time like any other

9. How do you think of the older years to be?

    J.   A time of growth and new experience

    B.   A time of despair and conflict

    C.   A static, nonproductive time

    E.   A time like any other

10. What is your general attitude toward aging?

    B. Afraid of it

    C. Resentful of it

    H. Eager for it

    I. Simply accept it

Scoring

Here's how to score your quiz:

1. Write in the letter for each answer in the "Letter" column.

2. Using the "Letter Values" list, find the value of points for each letter and write that number in the "Points" column.

3. Add up the points and write the total in the corresponding space.

4. Write in the *number of answers* you responded to for the section in the corresponding space, and divide that number into the sum of points.

The result is your self-image true age!

Letter Values

A = 5 B = 15 C = 25 D = 35 E = 45 F = 55 G = 65 H = 75 I = 85 J = 95

Self-Image True Age		
	Letter	Points
1.		
2.		
3.		
4.		
5.		
6.		
7.		
8.		
9.		
10.		
Total		
÷ #?s		
AQ		

Interpreting Your Score

An accurate reflection of who and what you are isn't carved in stone. It allows for fluctuations, growth, and changes. It has to. After all, self-image begins in childhood, as soon as one begins to comprehend how cute, smart, or mischievous he or she is. It continues to grow right through the teen years, young adulthood, midlife, and the autumnal years. A healthy self-image never stops growing and changing and maturing, just like a healthy individual never stops growing and changing and maturing. It is desirable to have a mature self-image, so if your AQ here is over 60, you're definitely going in the right direction.

Roles People Play

In social science circles, Karl Eisdorfer's "amoeba concept" has become a colorful tool illustrating the roles you play in life. An amoeba is an ever-changing organism influenced by nutrients and outside environmental factors—just like people. When it is well nourished and placed in a compatible environment, it is resilient, enduring, and malleable.

But removed from healthful sustenance, it dries out. Likewise, your environment must provide you with all the nutrients in order for you to be resilient, enduring, and malleable. What are the nutrients of your environment? They are the many roles you play: citizen, student, worker, spouse, lover, parent, child, friend, and so on.

At the center of these roles is a nucleus, the self. If you were to lose all your roles, you would dry up like the amoeba. Although these various roles needn't always be the same ones—in fact, they may shift frequently—they must be *there!* Too few, and your identity is on thin ice. Too many and the nucleus may be sated and overwhelmed. It is a delicate balance.

There are horrifying yet courageous stories of people who have surmounted incredible losses: amputees, paralysis victims, people who have had their entire families wiped out in an accident, people who, in Rudyard Kipling's words, "saw the things they gave their lives to broken, and stooped, and built 'em up with worn-out tools." These tales stir what is finest in us, because these brave people made a choice—a choice for life. They lost something great, but in the losing, they saw there were choices to be made, new roles to assume. The richness of their many roles enabled them to deal with their losses without ultimately drifting into a sea of confusion or conformity.

Wisdom of the Ages

A 39-year-old doctor gave up a lucrative practice to open a cooperative clinic where fees were based on ability to pay. Hiking Mount Shasta in northern California one year, a rock avalanche instantly killed his girlfriend. He was in a coma for five months. The doctors said it was futile, that if he came out of the coma, he would be in a vegetative state. Miraculously, he did come out of the coma, but he was in very bad shape. After a year of therapy, he was able to hold his head up, was learning to walk on crutches, and, using a spelling board, could keep a rapid-fire conversation going. He continued to be active with his clinic in whatever capacity he could. Rather than become bitter about his tragedy, he chose to view it as a conduit to greater learning and understanding—of himself, of the cosmos.

Fortunately, few suffer such cataclysms. But everyone suffers some kind of loss at one time or another. Even having to move from a neighborhood to which you've been accustomed can be a tremendous adjustment. Having a first child, or a second, completely changes who and what you are. You are gaining a new role (parent), but losing another. And when your children grow and leave home, you are losing a role (you are still the parent, of course, but no longer are you the guardian, police officer, and judge of their actions).

When a role is cut away from you—whether it's a role as a talking person, a working person, or a married person—you need to develop a new role. The strength for such accomplishment comes from self-knowledge. The better your understanding of who and what you are, the better you are able to fashion a full life.

As we mature, the roles we play change and become more complex. From the relative simplicity of adolescence to the coming of physical maturity in young adulthood and, hopefully, emotional maturity in middlescence, one experiences a second coming of maturity, a maturity of mind. It is the second brink of internal growth. As Jung described it, it is a time when people turn away from their concern with other people's opinions to concern with the growth of the self.

Self-Reflections

A great way to check up on your self-image AQ is to make a series of lists that reflect, in a very concrete way, who you are. These lists will help you raise your self-awareness and solidify your self-image AQ. The first of these four lists is an inventory of those elements that comprise your core being:

Priorities	Values	Fears	Fantasies
___	___	___	___
___	___	___	___
___	___	___	___
___	___	___	___

Under each heading, write whatever comes into your head. For example, under "priorities" you might list family, faith, and work. Under "values" you might list candor, honesty, compassion, and trustworthiness. When it comes to fears, a lot of folks will first write "losing a loved one"; but there are lots more. You might be terrified of heights, water, or poverty. Fantasies are a fun list and can include anything from an African safari to diving for buried treasure.

The lists can be as long as you wish. If you need more space than what's provided here, use a separate sheet of paper. Don't try to prioritize. Just get it all down first. After you've jotted down everything you can think of, rank each item in the order of importance to you.

Now grab a pad of paper and a pencil and take a few minutes to describe your distinct personality traits from your vantage point—how you see yourself.

Having trouble coming up with descriptions? Answering these questions might help. Are you …

- Bright and alert? Open-minded and adaptable?

- A loner, set in your ways, not too keen on what goes on around you?

- Shy or outgoing? Warm and friendly? Cautious and aloof?

- High energy, physically active, or quiet and contained?

- Garrulous or reticent? Lenient or judgmental?

- A good listener? Receptive to others' ideas?

- Opinionated? Assertive? Or passive, withdrawn?

Again, the list can be as long as you wish. If, as you continue to read this chapter, something else occurs to you, go ahead and add to it.

A reflection of your physical traits can be a real eye-opener when it comes to self-image:

- Do you stand tall, or do you stoop?

- Do you walk with confidence or in a halting manner?

♦ Do you have a big, open smile or a close-mouthed smile?

♦ Is your silhouette appealing, or are you too fat, too skinny, too lumpy?

♦ What is your usual expression—one of consternation, joy, thoughtfulness?

Perhaps you haven't thought about yourself in this way before. All the more reason to do so now. Look at yourself in the mirror and make an honest appraisal of what you see.

Finally, make a list of what you think the outside world sees when it looks at you:

♦ A person fastidious in appearance, ultra-casual, or sloppy?

♦ One who dresses fashionably, conservatively, or flamboyantly? Someone who is always tasteful in her attire, or someone who doesn't give a hoot about it?

♦ A person who takes a great deal of care in the appearance of his home, or one whose things are scattered helter-skelter? Do others see a welcoming home?

♦ If you have a car, how will others see a reflection of you in its appearance? Is it shiny and new? Old but pridefully kept up? Does it look like a neglected heap?

The answer to these and many other questions will help you develop an accurate self-image AQ. They will help you raise your self-awareness, enabling you to make changes in yourself. These tools allow for a realistic look at who and what you are. With a firm grip on that picture, you will better understand the dynamics in all your relationships.

Raising Up the Self-Image

Now that you've made your lists, you can take the next step. Imagine yourself in a variety of recent social settings—dinner last night, that party last week, the office this morning. Try to remember specific situations—pleasant ones, difficult ones, humorous ones, etc. Reflect on your behavior in the given situation.

Were you at ease or were you self-conscious? Were you comfortable enough to be genuine in the given situation, or did you camouflage your true self for fear that you wouldn't be accepted? Did you act bossy or meek, garrulous or reticent? Do you feel you were "the real you"?

How Many Candles?

Brought up in a small, southern city, this man loves the outdoors and now lives in the country. His work in sales demands that he travel a good deal; while it provides him with an excellent income, he thinks often about changing his line of work (financial AQ 56). Once divorced, he now maintains a good relationship with a woman, though they keep their own homes (significant other AQ 35). He is fit, trim, and physically active, as shown by his medical AQ of 35 and physical fitness AQ of 27. His sexuality AQ of 22 is a bit youngish for his years. Despite his Methodist upbringing, he is not religious, but is deeply spiritual (spiritual AQ 75). Upon examining himself in the mirror, he felt he looked worse than he expected. Yet he accepts with grace this time in his life, feeling it to be no better or worse than any other. He faces the future undauntingly (future AQ 76) and has a strong self-image AQ of 62. His true age is 50. His chronological age: 54. Good health and physical fitness will almost always put one's true age at or lower than one's chronological age when in midlife.

You may sometimes find yourself in a situation where you have to adapt your behavior in a way that may not be entirely comfortable. A tendency to be authoritative, for example, will likely be suppressed when you're taking orders from the boss. Or, despite some shyness and insecurity, you may find yourself in a leadership situation where you must appear to be authoritative. These are perfectly appropriate behavioral adaptations. But if you're constantly finding yourself having to push down parts of yourself, especially if it's to the point where the "real you" feels invisible, you're going to feel out of balance. You're going to begin to lose contact with who you are. That is an important clue, telling you to reconsider a variety of things: What kind of work are you doing? Can you be true to yourself on the job? What kind of friends have you made? Does their companionship encourage the true you to come out? Can you change any of these relationships? You want to find a way to reaffirm and support your sense of self.

So much of the doubt and anxiety that may plague you is an internal-ization of your earliest experiences, how you were seen by your parents and your siblings. As you grow and mature, whether knowingly or not, you often exhibit behavior based on these early internalizations, which can be childish, and even infantile. Over time, if you work at it, you can alter and shift some of those early beliefs. With growing self-awareness comes the ability to be self-actualizing, helping you to fully become the person you are.

Maintaining your integrity and sense of self is an on-going process. In the struggle to do so, you may very well lose the approval of some people in your life. But you will gain approval and acceptance of others. The friends and associates with whom you can be yourself are the ones worth keeping, for they unconditionally allow you to be who you are. There will always be those who demand that you be overly accommo-dating, who tit-for-tat and stroke-for-stroke you, who don't want their apple carts upset or the wheels of intimacy set in motion. Sometimes, in business, those relationships must be maintained. But it is important to see them for what they are. Don't fool yourself.

A youthful-looking woman in her 50s who does comedy gigs at local clubs butters her bread doing other work that helps support her pas-sion. She said, "I'm a lot older than I look. People are always shocked to find out my real age, not because I look so young, but because they think, 'Wow you really haven't done much with your life if you're that old, have you?'" She doesn't flinch. She may not have achieved fame and glory or made millions, but she's doing what she loves. She hasn't allowed such judgments to cause self-doubt. She's doing what she con-siders vital to herself. She has a strong self-image.

When you seek out those things that you really respond to, rather than passively accepting whatever is there, you are revitalizing your core being. What kind of literature comes into your home in the way of magazines and books? What television shows do you watch? Allowing the TV set or radio to run day and night with pure pap works against individuality. Conscious choices need to be made. Even eating habits can develop your uniqueness: Do you assemble menus based on your well-being, or are you going along with the tide of easy-to-prepare, readily available, overly processed and refined fast foods? Are you dis-tinctive in your choice of clothes, or do you scramble to purchase and parade about in the latest fashion?

Do you like being by yourself? One 55-year-old woman said, "I don't know if too many people like themselves the way I like myself, but I really do. I always have. I like myself so much that I enjoy my own company—I know that sounds weird, but there it is."

It doesn't sound the least bit weird. But in today's hustle bustle, when there's so much scurrying about in a social whirl that can leave you exhausted, it's rare to find that person who enjoys his own company, away from "the madding crowd." That doesn't make you a loner. A loner isn't necessarily a person who enjoys his own company. A loner may be a person who can't abide the company of others because he is filled with self-loathing: what one thinks of others is often a projection of what one thinks of himself. Enjoying your own company is essential to a mature self-image age quotient.

Changes and Expectations

A lot of people experience change as a crisis event: they panic and freeze, block and retreat. But no matter how clever their ploys, no matter how fast they run, they can't avoid change. It's part of the nature of things. Why not learn to greet change, to welcome it as the gateway to new adventures, new lessons, and new challenges?

Molding and shaping your life's pattern is an opportunity to which each of you is entitled. And it starts with the concept that you have of yourself. If you see yourself as capable, then the probability is that you will be capable. However, if you see yourself as incompetent, you will not, in all likelihood, develop your potential. If you believe that as a middle-aged person, it is too late for you to learn computer technology, for instance, it is unlikely you will learn it. If becoming a grandparent makes you think you've lost your youth, then you will have lost it.

On the other hand, if you believe you have undying energy and are up for taking on a new project, chances are you will do it. If you believe your mind is capable of learning a new language, you probably can. If you believe that your grandchildren offer you the opportunity to play creatively, as you haven't since your own childhood, then you will, in all likelihood, play creatively—and have a ball doing it! Some of these goals may take awhile, but where's the fire? Always appreciate every inch of progress you make, and be proud.

Events that elicit praise—getting a raise, earning a diploma, losing weight, becoming a grandparent—are exciting and rewarding because you get a lot of strokes from those around you, and that feels good. But praise is short-lived. People forget that you quit smoking, that you passed the state realtor's exam, that you built that greenhouse yourself, that you were promoted to supervisor. It's your own knowledge of these accomplishments, your own awareness of the original commitment and the strength it took to follow through, that promotes the kind of deep pride that raises your self-esteem.

A self-image must be cohesive if it is to hold together under duress. Be realistic in your self-appraisal, but be demanding; be kind, but don't be indulgent; be fastidious, but be open. Because you "don't" doesn't mean you "can't." A limited self-vision conditions you to living down to stifling expectations; an open-minded image equips you to living up to your full potential.

The attitudes developed and maintained toward age in general have a strong effect on your self-image AQ. While you may arrogantly deny or ignore this in your 20s and 30s, refusing to adapt appreciative attitudes toward your elders and the aging process will have an impact on you later on. If you see aging—whether physical, mental, or emotional—as a handicap, you place limitations on yourself that will be ultimately self-defeating.

Change is an integral part of life; it will come, whether or not it's invited. The changing roles you play, and your realistic self-appraisal and expectations, can help keep the nutrients of your environment healthy and thriving.

Acceptance

Self-image is at the root of how you perceive all your life experiences. It is important to work toward accepting yourself, to value yourself for your own intrinsic worth as a human being, not for what you have accomplished or impressed others with, but just for your own true self. Without self-acceptance, it is impossible to have a strong self-image. The process of learning self-acceptance is on-going and requires daily application.

What does self-acceptance mean? It allows you to be vulnerable, to have faults. Remember, you are not loved for being perfect. In all likelihood, it is your very imperfections, your idiosyncrasies, that make you loveable.

Self-acceptance demands that you embrace your curiosity, your child-like awe and daring. It also demands that you accept the "elder within," the one who is wise and patient. When the "elder within" coexists with your "inner child" and your present self, you will stand upon the springboard of a mature self-image AQ.

The way to acceptance is through positive thought patterns. Dr. Ronald Bennett of the Longevity Center says, "We're finding out more and more that the entire body chemistry can be changed with thought patterns, with how you think. It has an actual reaction on the physiological body." In other words, if you think angry thoughts, a chemical reaction begins that has an intense reaction on your body. If you think passionate thoughts, likewise, a chain of chemical reactions is set off. Research has shown that the most beneficial chemical bath you can give yourself is created by having compassionate and peaceful thoughts.

Learning to be compassionate with yourself and to respect each important aspect of your self—your body, your sexuality, your health, your work, your recreation, your relationships, your communication skills—will lead you to self-acceptance, resulting in a strong self-image AQ. A solid, nonlimiting, mature self-image has far-reaching and positive effects that can give you the power and flexibility needed to navigate your way through the sea of life.

A clear, bold look in the looking glass of your own soul, and in the reflection of the eyes of your families, friends, and coworkers, is what it takes. It may seem frightening, but it's an exciting adventure. Remember the turtle: she never makes progress unless she sticks her neck out.

The Least You Need to Know

- Self-awareness requires realistic self-analysis.
- It's easier to deal with change and loss when you have many roles in life.
- Reflections of how others see you raise your self-awareness.
- Positive expectations reinforce an "I can" attitude.
- Self-acceptance is vital to a strong self-image.

Chapter 8

Spirituality True Age

In This Chapter

- ◆ Optimizing your spiritual true age
- ◆ Discovering various pathways to your higher self
- ◆ Adopting rituals and celebrations
- ◆ Assembling the essential ingredients to spiritual practice
- ◆ Learning to be grateful

In the past, the very marrow of spiritual life was one's church or temple. At least once a week, everyone put on his or her Sabbath finery to join the community for a lesson in and reminder of the spiritual side of life. That still holds true today for many people, but for many others, while spirituality still plays an important part in their lives, it is often in a less traditional way.

Your Spiritual True Age Quiz

1. How do you celebrate birthdays and anniversaries?

   I. Every year with friends and relatives

   H. Every year with one special friend

   G. Every other year or so with friends and relatives

   F. Every other year or so with one special friend

   D. I don't celebrate these events

2. How do you celebrate national holidays (Thanksgiving, Fourth of July, etc.)?

   I. Every year with friends and relatives

   H. Every year with one special friend

   G. Every other year or so with friends and relatives

   F. Every other year or so with one special friend

   D. I don't celebrate these events

3. How do you celebrate religious holidays like Christmas, Easter, Passover, Ramadan, or Kwanza?

   I. Every year with friends and relatives

   H. Every year with one special friend

   G. Every other year or so with friends and relatives

   F. Every other year or so with one special friend

   D. I don't celebrate these events

4. If you are affiliated with a church or synagogue, how often do you attend? (Note, if you are not affiliated, do not answer this question.)

   I. Regularly, on a weekly basis

   F. Once or twice a month

   D. On special occasions, like holidays or other celebrations

   A. Rarely

5. Do you get solace from your spiritual path?

    G. A great deal

    F. Some

    D. On occasion

    B. Not at all

6. Do you meditate or pray?

    J. On a daily basis

    H. A few times a week

    D. Only when there's a special need

    B. Not at all

7. How do you feel about your spiritual life?

    J. It is mostly rich and full.

    B. I feel an emptiness inside.

    C. It's not something I'm concerned about.

    F. I haven't found the right path yet, but I'm searching.

    E. It ebbs and flows.

8. How do you feel about humankind?

    J. Good or bad, we're all interconnected.

    C. I don't think about it.

    G. There are good people and bad people; I'll go with the good ones.

    D. Everyone's out for himself.

9. Which of the following choices best reflects your own attitude or philosophy?

    D. The doctrines of my faith.

    G. Nature itself is supreme.

    G. There is only one Supreme Being.

    H. There is a unity of all life.

    G. There is no Supreme Being.

    G. There is something greater than me but I don't know what it is.

    C. I don't think about it.

10. What is your attitude about humankind's relationship to the planet?

   J. We are all stewards of the earth.

   B. I don't think about it.

   C. Take care of your own backyard.

   D. It's government's responsibility.

   E. It's in the hands of the corporate world.

   F. Nothing we do will alter the course of nature.

Scoring

Here's how to score your quiz:

1. Write in the letter for each answer in the "Letter" column.

2. Using the "Letter Values" box, find the value of points for each letter and write that number in the "Points" column.

3. Add up the points and write the total in the corresponding space.

4. Write in the *number of answers* you responded to for the section in the corresponding space, and divide that number into the sum of points.

The result is your spirituality true age!

Letter Values

A = 5 B = 15 C = 25 D = 35 E = 45 F = 55 G = 65 H = 75 I = 85 J = 95

	Letter	Points
Spirituality True Age		
1.		
2.		
3.		
4.		
5.		
6.		
7.		
8.		
9.		
10.		
Total		
÷ #?s		
AQ		

Interpreting Your Score

When it comes to your spiritual AQ, a mature score is indicative of deep spirituality. In no way does your spiritual AQ depend upon how active you are with an organized religion. Whether you're 20 or 40, a score of 60 or 70 is entirely within the realm of possibility, no matter what your religious affiliation. Of course, a high AQ here will raise your true age. But, as the entire thesis of this book has set out to prove, "older" is not bad, just as "younger" is not necessarily good. It all depends on context. If you are a person who doesn't give a hoot about your spiritual life and you end up with a young spiritual AQ, so be it. There are no judgments here, just assessments.

If your church or temple is the central part of your spiritual life, it is probably also a central part of your social life. Church picnics and bake-offs, weekly choir practice, Sunday school, even family camps, can evolve from a religious center. But there has been a gradual falling away from organized religion as a social and spiritual core on the part of many. Some believe this falling away is responsible for a lowering of values and the eradication of certain social mores. However, where there are appropriate alternatives for organized religion in one's life, spiritual values and mores need not be lowered, though they may change. They may even be elevated.

What Is Spirituality?

In *Zen in the Art of Archery*, author Eugen Herrigel writes, "For master archers, it is a fact of common experience that a good archer can shoot further with a medium-strong bow than an unspiritual archer can with the strongest. It does not depend on the bow, but on the presence of mind, on the vitality and awareness with which you shoot." A healthy acceptance and appreciation of your perpetual becoming will help you to shoot straight and far, even if your bow isn't quite as strong as it once was. This is especially true because, just as each of you possesses many ages, each of you possesses many strengths, the physical being only one—and the simplest one, at that.

Here is where education can come into play: attending classes, lectures, and seminars aimed at the finer side of life. The arts, philosophy, meditation, spirituality, nature, ecology, and subjects geared toward the godhead, the cosmos, or universality can become an excellent alternative for organized religion insofar as spiritual growth is concerned.

Unitarian Universalist minister Frances West says, "Human beings have a desire to worship because it scratches what itches in the human condition." Most people feel a longing for something beyond the mere act of survival. Everyone wants love, connection, relationship. You get much of that from your family, your friends, and your community. But there is a stronger itch in many, an itch for some understanding of the greatness and vastness of this universe in which we are but tiny specks.

Most of you have experienced, at least once in your lifetime, a singular moment of connectivity with the cosmos. A moment when you truly felt at one with the world, that you were, indeed, an integral part of the universe. Those moments—moments that take your breath away—are the flint stones that ignite the fire of life. Think about those moments in your life when the sparks lit up everything around you:

♦ A baby reaching up to touch your cheek

◆ The first time you said "I love you" to someone who wasn't a member of your family

◆ Seeing the sky on a crisp, clear night, 100 miles from the nearest city or town

◆ Watching a flock of white pelicans appear and disappear as they dip and swoop across the sky

◆ Hearing your child's first word

The list could go on and on, and it alone would more than adequately make the point that spirituality is the innermost core of your being: deeper than love, deeper than self-image. It is the common thread that binds all humans. Everyone recognizes themselves in these experiences.

Ask yourself, what are the sights, sounds, smells, touches, tastes, actions, silence, words, and motions you remember? What was the itch that got scratched? Write them down.

Wisdom of the Ages

A little boy packed his suitcase with Twinkies and a six-pack of root beer and started off on a journey to meet God. About three blocks from home, he saw an elderly man sitting in the park feeding some pigeons. The boy sat down next to him. He thought the man looked hungry, so he offered him a Twinkie. The man gratefully accepted it and smiled at the boy. His smile was so pleasant, the boy offered him a root beer. Again, the man smiled at him. The boy was delighted! All afternoon they sat eating and smiling, but they never said a word.

As it grew dark, the boy got up to leave. He had gone just a few steps, when he turned around, ran back, and gave the old man a hug. The man gave him his biggest smile ever.

Seeing the look of joy on the boy's face when he got home, his mother asked, "What did you do today that made you so happy?" He replied, "I had lunch with God. You know what? God's got the most beautiful smile I've ever seen!"

Meanwhile, the elderly man returned to his home. Stunned by the look of peace on his face, his son asked, "Dad, what did you do today that made you so happy?" He replied, "I ate Twinkies in the park with God. You know, he's much younger than I expected."

The Hierarchy of Needs

Abraham Maslow, the father of humanistic psychology, set forth a theory in 1943 that has become widely accepted today. The hierarchy of human needs proposes that an individual is ready to act upon the higher needs if and only if some basic needs are met. He theorized that these basic needs are physiological health, safety, love, affection, a sense of belonging, and self-esteem. When these needs are met, one feels self-confident and valuable as a person in the world. When these needs are frustrated, the person feels inferior, weak, helpless, and worthless.

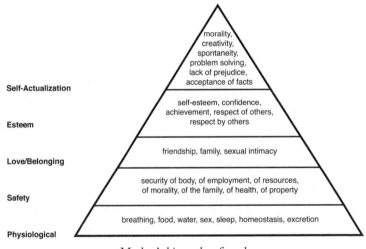

Maslow's hierarchy of needs.

He set these needs up in a pyramid. Once the basic first four needs are met, Maslow suggested, the person can proceed up the pyramid to the higher needs of self-actualization. Self-actualized people are characterized by the following:

- Being problem-focused

- Incorporating an ongoing freshness of appreciation of life

- A concern about personal growth

- The ability to have peak experiences (such as those listed in the "What Is Spirituality?" section)

In later years, Maslow differentiated the growth needs of self-actualization, breaking it down into even more levels:

◆ **Cognitive** to know, to understand, and explore

◆ **Aesthetic** symmetry, order, and beauty

◆ **Self-actualization** to find self-fulfillment and realize one's potential

◆ **Transcendence** to connect to something beyond the ego or to help others find self-fulfillment and realize their potential

Everyone whose basic needs are satisfied begins to look beyond the immediate. The search for wholeness, unity, integration, oneness—these are the essentials of the spiritual experience. The desire to see justice in the world, the search for truth and orderliness, to feel a sense of belonging to the universe, to be a world citizen—these, too, are a part of spirituality. To find your own inner essence, to practice spirituality by meditation and by your actions, to be authentic and stay pure in purpose—this is spirituality.

How Many Candles?

She lives in a London flat with her significant other, far from her Michigan roots. The two have a solid relationship (significant other AQ 44). She earns a decent living as a campaign initiative assistant, a job she's very satisfied with, and feels confident of advancement (financial AQ 53). Her physical fitness AQ is 39, and would be lower if she exercised more often and got a little more sleep. She has a rewarding circle of friends but not enough time to enjoy leisure activities (social AQ 53). Though she isn't religious, she feels deeply spiritual and enjoys celebrating holidays and rituals with friends and family (family AQ 68). Open to change, comfortable with the pace of life, she welcomes new challenges (future AQ 85).

Her true age is 54. Her chronological age: 24. Her maturity has boosted her true age in a positive way, but her sluggish physical fitness and lack of balance in leisure time activities has boosted it higher than it needs to be. Some work in these areas is recommended.

Your values reflect your judgment about what is important in life. Maslow suggested a list of values that are important in defining one's being; he called them B Values. Rather than quickly scanning this long list, try saying each word aloud to yourself, allowing two or three seconds of reflection after each line.

- Wholeness/Unity/Oneness
- Perfection/Just-so-ness
- Completion/Finality/Ending
- Justice/Fairness
- Aliveness/Full-Functioning
- Richness/Intricacy
- Simplicity/Essential/Honesty
- Beauty/Form/Richness
- Goodness/Oughtness
- Uniqueness/Idiosyncrasy/Novelty
- Effortlessness/Ease/Perfect
- Playfulness/Joy/Humor
- Truth/Reality/Beauty/Pure
- Self-Sufficiency/Independence

Each of these values is worthy of focused contemplation and practice.

Maslow believed that education was key to assisting people toward growth. He had a great deal of advice for educators to aid them in encouraging individuals to reach their full potential as self-actualized people. Among his instructions were teaching people to focus on the right career and the right mate, to appreciate beauty and nature, to understand their inner selves, to be open to joy, and to transcend their cultural conditions and become world citizens.

The Practice of Spirituality

Spirituality is a practice. It doesn't just happen. You have to work at it, like anything worthwhile. The soul will not take care of itself if you do not take care of it. It's the same as saying, "I wish I could write," and not trying it, every day, month after month, over and over again; or, "I wish I could jog 5 miles a day," and, when you can't even jog 1 mile, giving up and saying, "I can't do it." Or like saying, "I wish I liked this place" without working at being mindful of all the many things there are to like about it.

Each of you is as unique in your spirituality as you are in your footprints. The path to freedom—and that is what inner balance and harmony is—is a personal, individualistic quest that leads to greater and greater clarity, openness, and vision. It cannot be taken under the guise of someone else's journey, someone who lived 5,000 years ago or 1,000 years ago or 500 years ago, or is living now. It has to be your journey, your insight, your footprint.

There are so many paths that can assist you in your quest, it's hard to choose or find the "right" one. There may be no right one; there may be many. Investigate. Explore. Experience. Dig in.

Rituals and Celebrations

Rituals and ceremonies add meaning and purpose to life events. They help you embrace change. They help you express important emotions, including love and grief. They help build community. And they enhance personal connections with the spirit of life itself. What rituals or celebrations have been most memorable to you?

In addition to all the obvious rituals people generally celebrate—birthdays, anniversaries, graduations, religious and national holidays—there are other times and events that often go unheeded in life, yet they lend themselves splendidly to creating ritual and celebration.

- For girls, the onset of menses
- For boys, his first shave or change of voice

- The first budding of roses in spring

- The first snowfall in winter

- The reunion of family or friends after being apart

Creating ritual is, simply, creating structure, some kind of formal act or ceremony that marks the occasion. For example, friends could establish retreats with each other, a day or two or more entirely devoted to baring each other's soul to one another, reading inspiring passages aloud, taking long walks. Or families and neighbors could do a potluck, sharing food and libations to celebrate the first flowering of spring. These rituals enrich one's spiritual journey and strengthen bonds between family members, friends, and neighbors.

Prayers and Blessings

When a person sneezes, you often hear someone around her say, "Gesundheit!" This is a German word meaning "good health." To say "Gesundheit" is to bless someone. It isn't necessary to be a preacher or a cleric to bless others. It is only necessary to be sincere.

When blessings are created for daily routines, you make of them a ritual. If at dinnertime the family joins hands for a moment of silence, that is a ritual. Or, if a member of the family speaks a prayer of thanksgiving before meals, that is a ritual.

Optimize Your AQ

Why not create blessings for special occasions in your life? If your child is giving her first piano recital, before she goes on stage, hold her hands and say, "Bless these hands, that they may be steadfast and nimble, following the path you have taught them so well." If your husband is going in for heart surgery, place your hands on his heart and say, "Bless this heart, so sure and strong, that has given me so much strength over the years. May my heart's strength flow into yours in these next hours."

Many people think they don't pray, or they pray only in church. But when you are in difficult straits and impulsively cry out, "Oh, god, please, I don't know if I can handle this," that is a form of prayer. When someone you love is sick or injured and you wish very hard for their recovery, that is prayer. If you are lost in the woods, you pray for some sign to help you find your way out. If you find some formal opening and closing to these spontaneous prayers, you will be ritualizing them. By so doing, you will stay more focused on what you want, what you need, thus bringing more meaning to your prayers and to yourself.

Meditation

Meditation is a practice of reflection and contemplation. It's different than prayer. You might think of it as a kind of music, or an art form, or a play within a play.

Thinking of the practice of meditation as music, we suggest that it is not classical music: it's jazz. A different tune with different riffs every day. You get to make it up as you go along. Like any music, it takes practice. And the more you practice, the richer and fuller the sound you produce. Thinking of the practice of meditation as a painting, we suggest not realistic, but abstract art, and a different canvas every day. You get to make it up as you go along. Like any art, it takes practice. And the more you practice, the more exquisite the image.

Thinking of the practice of meditation as a play, we suggest improvisational theatre, rather than a set piece. Every day is different, ad libbed. You get to make it up as you go along. And the more you practice, the more likely you are to achieve a memorable creation.

Some people like to have a special place in their home or garden to meditate, and perhaps some special icon to place before them, which helps to keep them focused: a tree, a rock, a statue, a painting. Appropriate background music can be helpful, too. Taking time out of your busy day to practice your spirituality is a splendid ritual.

Optimize Your AQ

You can practice mindful living at anytime, in any place. Right now, take two minutes to appreciate the feel of this book in your hands. Sit back. Take a deep breath or two and glory in the miracle of your lungs and body. Look around you. Smell, feel, taste. See colors, textures, shapes, quality of light, ambiance.

But not everybody likes or is able to practice on a daily basis. It takes up too much time. It gets boring. Here's a way you can incorporate meditation with the simplest, most daily routine tasks. Each of the following can be the structure within which you meditate:

◆ Washing dishes: the focus is on cleansing and renewal

◆ Folding laundry: the focus is on order and accomplishment

◆ Making the bed: the focus is on chaos and order

◆ Taking a bath: the focus is on healing and relaxation

◆ Washing your hands: the focus is on ability and achievement

The important thing is to practice.

Gratitude

Part of the practice of spirituality is learning and remembering to be grateful for what you have in your life. Even during the worst of times, there is always something to be grateful for. Before you go to bed or after you arise in the morning, do a simple review of all that you have to be grateful for in the last 24 hours. It may include a good night's sleep, a delicious meal, or a good laugh.

This quick, simple method will help you remember the great store of moments and events each day has to offer. You don't want your life to fly by in a blur. Kierkegaard once said, "We live life forward but understand it backward." A brief review such as this affords an understanding and insight quite different than that which you experience while in the midst of the doing.

Practicing any or all of these techniques will surely lead to a very mature spirituality AQ.

Finding Your Spiritual Path

There is no one path leading to spiritual enlightenment. There are many. Which is as it should be, considering the diversity of human sensibilities and intelligences. Some follow a single path all their lives, the same path their parents and grandparents followed. Others diverge only slightly from that path, while still others feel compelled to try every-thing, never settling on any one path.

Certainly the goal of any spiritual path is to be able to open your heart so that you can love and care for others. Pose these questions to your-self:

> How do you show care, love, and respect to yourself? To your family? To your friends? To your enemies?

The Chinese have a saying: "When you have 100 miles to travel, con-sider 90 half the journey." When it comes to your spiritual path, there really is no "there," no actual destination. It's all about being on a path, about having an active, seeking, beseeching spiritual journey.

In addition to the traditional religions with which you are all familiar, what are some of the paths that may seem more experimental to your culture? Here are a few:

- Hinduism, characterized by a belief in reincarnation and a supreme being that takes many forms and natures; Hindus seek liberation from earthly evils.

- Buddhism, which believes that suffering is inseparable from exis-tence and that spiritual enlightenment is beyond both suffering and existence. Zen Buddhism, an offshoot, is based on the practice of meditation.

- Wicca, a pagan nature-based religion.

- Totemism, a belief in the kinship and/or symbology of animals, plants, or natural objects.

- Pantheism, which relates to the entire universe as being identified with the godhead.

Any one of these paths have techniques and rituals that will stimulate spiritual thinking, from reading runes or the I-Ching, to commun-ing with trees and rocks, to acknowledging the diverse representations of god in nature. All these paths ultimately lead to the same things: mindful living, discovering your interconnectedness, humbling yourself before forces greater than yourself.

The late Rachel Carson once wrote, "The surf that you find exhilarating at Virginia Beach or at La Jolla today may have lapped at the base of antarctic icebergs or sparkled in the Mediterranean sun, years ago, before it moved through dark and unseen waterways to the place you find it now." She also wrote, "For all at last return to the sea—to Oceanus, the ocean river, like the ever-flowing stream of time, the beginning and the end."

The Least You Need to Know

- Because spirituality is a practice, you need to work at it every day.
- There are many paths that can guide you along the path to your higher self.
- Meditation and prayer are an integral part of any spiritual practice.
- Reviewing each day and noting what you're grateful for leads to greater self-understanding and insight.
- Spirituality is the search for your higher self.

Chapter 9

Future True Age

In This Chapter

- Optimizing your future true age
- Adapting to change
- Continuing your education
- Planning for the future
- Examining expectations

No matter what age you are, you are among the aging. Although the maturation of the physical body reaches its peak at about 25 or 30, at which point it begins a very gradual decline (how gradual is, in great part, up to you), intellectually, spiritually, and emotionally. You can continue to grow toward peak periods until your last days. Your future AQ depends on how well you adapt to change, continue learning, and plan for the future, the subjects of this chapter.

Your Future True Age Quiz

1. What do you seek to accomplish in the future?

    H. I hope to realize goals set during my youth.

    I.   I hope to figure out new goals and realize them.

    F. I want to put aside ambition, to relax and enjoy.

    B. I just want to get through it. Forget goals!

2. What have you done in the recent past and what do you plan to do in the near future to add to your education or skills?

    B. Nothing in particular.

    H. I have learned a new skill (e.g., language, carpentry, computer programming).

    J.   I have acquired a college degree or other professional credential (e.g., realtor's license, mediator's certificate).

    G. Nothing tangible, but I am constantly reading and trying to educate myself.

3. How does recreational activity fit into your life plan?

    B. It doesn't; I consider it a waste of time.

    I.   It is a regular and frequent part of my life.

    D. I only indulge on holidays and vacations.

    E. I participate only occasionally, but strive to do so more often.

4. How do you feel about the rate of speed with which the technological world is changing?

    H. A little fast, but I keep up

    B. Too fast for me

    I.   Just about the right pace

    J.   A little slow for my tastes

    C. Too slow; I get bored

5. When you experience a positive but dramatic change in your life (new job, moving, etc.), what feelings most frequently accompany those changes?

   J. Excitement, an adventurous feeling

   B. Depression, restless moodiness

   C. Anxiety, a threatening feeling

   H. Acceptance

6. How do you feel about modern technology?

   G. It's exciting and wonderful.

   J. It's useful, but it can also be harmful.

   D. It's gotten way ahead of us.

   F. There's more than we need or want.

   A. It's beyond my understanding.

   E. It's exciting but overwhelming.

7. If and when you retire, what will your income earning capacity do?

   I. It will gradually increase.

   C. It will gradually decrease.

   D. It will remain the same, but without cost-of-living increases.

   H. It will remain the same with regular cost-of-living increases.

   B. It will be very unpredictable.

8. How would you compare your life experiences with the expectations of your youth?

   J. Very fulfilling

   G. Somewhat fulfilling

   H. Expectations have radically changed

   C. Rather unfulfilling

9. How has the death of someone close to you made you feel?

    B. That life has no meaning

    J. That time is precious and I want to use it well

    C. Abandoned and alone

    E. Not much different from before

    C. Angry and short-changed

    A. Frightened for my life

10. What is your outlook toward the future?

    J. I approach it eagerly.

    B. It frightens me.

    H. Whatever it brings, I'll deal with it.

    D. I don't think about it much.

    C. I'd like things to stay as they are.

11. Under what circumstances would you be willing to pull up roots and move to another city?

    E. I'd go only if I had to (e.g., job transfer).

    B. I would not relocate under any circumstances.

    H. I'd go only if the move promised new challenges and opportunities.

    D. I'd go if the move represented a complete change in lifestyle; otherwise, why bother?

    C. I'd go in a minute; I don't like being in one place for long.

12. What kind of plans have you made for your own death?

    J. I have both a living will and a regular will, with instructions for my burial as well as distribution of my property.

    G. I have a regular will with instructions for distribution of my property.

    E. I don't have a will, but my family knows my wishes.

    B. I don't want to think about it.

Scoring

Here's how to score your quiz:

1.   Write in the letter for each answer in the "Letter" column.

2.   Using the "Letter Values" list, find the value of points for each letter and write that number in the "Points" column.

3   Add up the points and write the total in the corresponding space.

4.   Write in the *number of answers* you responded to for the section in the corresponding space and divide that number into the sum of points.

The result is your future true age!

Letter Values
A = 5 B = 15 C = 25 D = 35 E = 45 F = 55 G = 65 H = 75 I = 85 J = 95

	Future True Age	
	Letter	**Points**
1.		
2.		
3.		
4.		
5.		
6.		
7.		
8.		
9.		
10.		
11.		
12.		
Total		
÷ #?s		
AQ		

Interpreting Your Score

Adaptability means watching and listening to the changing world around you with an open mind. If you humbug every stroke of progress that comes along—whether it's hybrid cars, HDTV, or a new form of birth control—you'll become mired in the past, suffocating possibilities for growth. So when it comes to your future AQ, the most desirable outcome is a mature age. Even a young adult in her 20s can achieve an AQ of 60, 70, even 80 in this category. Sure, it will boost your overall true age, but that will be a mark of your maturity.

On the other hand, if your attitude about the changes you see in the world is largely negative—if you dig in your heels at the thought of trying something new—your future AQ will be very young indeed. That, in turn, will pull down your true age. A very young true age in an adult in his 50s or 60s is not necessarily a wonderful thing.

Dealing with Change

Futurist Alvin Toffler gave us the term "culture shock," which he defines as "the effect that immersion in a strange culture has on the unprepared visitor." For the unprepared, middle and old age—even early adulthood—may be just such a "strange culture," sending us into "age shock": You receive an invitation to attend the 20-year reunion of your high school graduating class. Twenty years? It can't be! Or you're discussing movie classics with a group of people when one of the younger fellows chimes in, "Geez, that's a really old movie." You look at him and say, "It's not that old—I saw it in college." Then you remember that you attended college before he was born. Age shock.

> **Wisdom of the Ages**
>
> In our rapidly changing society we can count on only two things that will never change. What will never change is ... the will to change and the fear of change.
>
> —Harriet Goldhor Lerner

The tendency to picture yourself as you were when you were young is widespread. While that is harmless—perhaps even helpful—if it's coupled with a fixed idea of who and what you are, you're going to suffer from age shock, for you're not going to be able to adapt. And adapting to change has everything to do with your future AQ.

A lot of people are no longer as flexible as they were at 20. They are less willing or able to roll with the punches life is constantly throwing at them. But the world is changing so rapidly, unless you take yourself out of the freezer and work at thawing out, you're going to remain frozen in the past.

Before and After

A good warm-up might be to review and update your "befores and afters." Everyone has these life-changing experiences: before Murray died, after Angela was born, before I got married, after I lost my job. You may have several of these trail markers, and keep adding to them. But for some, one or two pivotal times become fixed points signifying their only peak experiences—with the "after" being all on the downside. For one 31-year-old man, life had already peaked at 23. A high school football hero who managed a successful nightclub for a few years after graduation, to this day, those are his most animated topics of conversation. He eventually married, fathered two children, and divorced. He stays home much of the time, watches sports on TV, goes to a few rock concerts, and hates his job. Nothing interests him. At 31, he has no "befores" ahead of him because he puts no effort into creating anything new and stimulating for himself. Unless he breaks this pattern, the rest of his life will remain a waiting game.

Fear of change can virtually paralyze you, and yet change is a harbinger of growth. When computers began to take over the business world, everyone worried that the job market would shrink dramatically. What happened instead was that a whole new field opened up, one that required new skills. People trained and prepared themselves for this new technological era. Initially, some people did lose jobs, it's true, but many of them were catapulted into entirely new work experiences. If they didn't freeze up, the jolt completely revitalized their lives.

If you can keep your "befores and afters" updated and malleable, you'll be able to take stock of what you do and don't want to do with your life, and of what you can and cannot change. In other words, you may discover the active ingredients of both your discontent and your pleasure.

Optimize Your AQ

Establish new goals, but be realistic. If you're 39 years old and want to become a runner, forget the Olympics; but do begin a training program, which in a year or so will enable you to enter marathons. If you want your own business and you're 58, don't think "corporate empire": just start a small business in your home, one that will keep you active long after you've received the company gold watch.

Natural disasters can devastate the countryside. But given time, new growth will appear. It is much the same with personal loss and disaster. Mourning losses for an appropriate period is necessary and proper; but if you cling to your losses, you will stifle all potential for future development, growth, and creativity. Past events—whether losses or gains—can be used to cultivate the soil of your everyday life, ensuring a wholesome and abundant harvest. With an attitude like that, you're bound to have a mature future AQ.

Tools to Make Transitions

Change is unavoidable. The world is in a constant state of flux. You can try to blind yourself to it, try to stave it off, try to turn your back on it. But eventually you have to face it: Your company is transferring you to a new location. You're starting a brand new job. You're getting married. Your father is old and must move in with you and your family. There are ways of dealing with change that can make it easier.

In dealing with personal changes, it seems there are always three stages you have to go through:

1. Letting go
2. Dealing with uncertainty
3. Moving forward

Letting go: The first stage can be very hard because there may be a lot of emotion involved: you may have to leave people and places behind that you were very attached to. You may not feel ready to do so and resist the change. Here are some of the tools that can help you get through letting go:

♦ Acknowledge your past accomplishments.

- Acknowledge that those you leave behind can continue to be a support to you, even if they're not nearby.

- Express your feelings to the people you're leaving.

- Find some symbol of the places and things you're leaving to carry with you.

Resist getting nostalgic about what you're leaving behind. You will have fond memories, of course, but nostalgia is a way of sentimentalizing the past that can make it harder to walk into your future.

Dealing with uncertainty: Of course you are going to feel anxious and unsure. You're going into an entirely new situation. Who wouldn't be a little uneasy? Here are some techniques and tools to help you deal with uncertainty:

- Get as much accurate information as you can about every aspect of your forthcoming venture.

- Seek encouragement from those who believe in you.

- Do a self-assessment, acknowledging the strengths and skills you possess to make this transition.

- Be open and transparent about your uncertainties with friends and loved ones.

Moving forward: Once you've passed through these first two stages, you are ready to move forward. To make your transition as successful as possible, it helps to do the following:

- Create a mission statement for yourself, outlining what you aim to accomplish in your new city, your new job, your new relationship.

- Write down your expectations.

- Visit the places that will be helpful to you in your new endeavor.

- Ally yourself with one or two organizations that suit your interests and needs so that you may begin to form new connections.

In Chapters 13 and 15, you will learn a lot more about how to get connected to individuals and to your community.

How Many Candles?

A professor at a college in Fairbanks, Alaska, this Boston-born management expert has a close relationship with her second husband; they regularly share recreational activities and important decision-making (significant other AQ 41). A mother of three, a grandmother of four, and the eldest of four sisters, her family ties are very close-knit (family AQ 63). Physically fit (physical fitness AQ 24) and sharp as a tack (brain fitness AQ 38), she's deeply spiritual (spiritual AQ 71), though she doesn't consider herself religious. She is very interested in the political scene; while she votes in national and statewide elections, and contributes to causes, she is not particularly involved in community events and volunteers only occasionally: her community AQ is 50. Content staying put, big changes do make her feel somewhat anxious, but she deals well with technology and is constantly reading and learning (future AQ 50).

Her true age is 40. Her chronological age: 65. Her good health and fine physical fitness pulled her true age way down. If she was more involved in her community and less uncertain about change, it would probably have been closer to 50, a wonderful true age for any 65-year-old.

Making changes requires a lot of energy and concentration. It's important not to be impulsive about it. Impetuosity often ends in regret, causing you to be even more reluctant the next time you confront change. Because change always whips up a certain amount of stress, the smart approach is to break down the anticipated changes into as many small, separate steps as you can. This makes things a lot easier to handle.

Education: Your Key to the Future

Intellectual growth continues throughout adulthood for those who remain intellectually active. Unfortunately, for most of the population, a marked decline begins around the age of 25 because most people do not challenge their minds (see Chapter 6). Education doesn't necessarily mean school. Education simply means obtaining knowledge or a skill through a learning process. Education can mean the following:

♦ Reading with purpose rather than for entertainment

♦ Visiting a museum or art gallery and examining both the work and your responses to it

- ◆ Cultivating a garden
- ◆ Building a tree house
- ◆ Studying French in the comfort of your den

Whatever you undertake, you will be truly educating yourself if you do embark on your new adventure in a thorough manner. That means careful preparation, committed follow-through, and follow-ups. Education, whether formal or do-it-yourself, is a primary factor in removing the strictures that keep one from adapting to change.

Education should be an ongoing process, stretched out over a lifetime. There are myriad resources ensuring your ability to do that, including continuing education courses, professional development courses, computer training classes, and lessons in everything from dance to golf to first aid. Let your imagination run wild!

The list is long. There's so much available—and much of it is free! (See Chapter 14 for additional work-related resources.) There is just no good excuse for not keeping up; if you don't, you will make good the ageist term "old fogey."

Pursuing a hobby can be very educational, and offer a worthy activity you can continue to practice and enjoy long after your working life is past. Find something based on your very personal desires and delights. There is a hobby for every taste, whether it's collecting stamps, gardening, bird watching, or knitting.

Wisdom of the Ages

How the world must have been changing while I was holding it still.

—Tom Stoppard

Keeping up and keeping occupied keeps you vital. Vitality is the key to good living. Although vitality is associated with youth, there are an awful lot of young people who are most decidedly not filled with vitality. Vitality belongs to those who make an effort, who make the decision to adapt, and who fill their lives with purpose, education, and adventure.

Preparing for the Future

Some of you may never think about getting older; others may think of little else. In your younger years, you consider it fleetingly, if at all. But as you get older, you tend to think of it increasingly—sometimes with a good deal of trepidation. This is particularly so when a loved one falls fatally ill or dies.

It's important to plan for the future. But you don't want to be so busy planning for the future that when the future catches up with you, you're right back to planning for the future again. Living entirely for that presumed time to come will alienate you from the day-to-day world. It's vital to live in the here and now. But if you set goals for the future, and put things in place to ensure their success, the present will be a lot more constructive. And your anxiety about the future will be greatly reduced.

Just as education can dispel many fears and help you overcome obstacles, so can preparation for your later years remove much of the trepidation you may feel. Being entitled to Social Security at 65 will hardly mean that you're going to be taken care of. That doesn't mean you must put the bulk of today's time, energy, and money into a future destiny, but there are some practical measures that can and should be taken.

Securing Your Future

Now's the time to make sure that medical care will be available to you later on. Explore long-term care, Medicare, and supplemental plans. Learn everything you can about benefits accruing to you from pension plans and Social Security. You may discover, for example, that if you work just another eight months, your pension will go up markedly. Or you may find that you can "retire" from your company, take your pension, and continue doing work for the company as a consultant!

Do what you can to build a financial nest egg. Put something away every month—even if it's only a few bucks. It's a start!

Consider investing in a home of your own so you won't have to worry about a roof over your head when you're 75.

Consider whether or not you want to leave the traditional workplace by a certain age to pursue other interests. What might they be? Take stock. What excites and stimulates you? Develop a hobby, start a fitness program, plan a second career, initiate a small home business, or sharpen a new skill for part-time work. Think about how and where you want to live when you're older—with family, alone, in a retirement community? Talk to older people and ask them what it's like to be older. How did they prepare for their old age? What would they do differently? Not only will you be gaining valuable information, but you'll also be crossing the age gap that isolates older people from everyone else.

Planning the End

Unwelcome as it might be, it's wise to have a plan for your death. Prepare a will. You might want to hire a lawyer to help you with this task, or use one of the many estate-planning programs available online. If you have even modest holdings, you need to think about how you want them disbursed after you're gone. Review your expectations and desires. You might even want to leave some words of love and wisdom as a legacy. Not only will this bring great comfort and aide to those who survive you, but knowing your house is in order will comfort you in the here and now. By giving it a little thought now, you will not be pressed to make such considerations at a time when you might not have the clarity of thought or the energy.

Having a will saves your family needless anguish when you die, no matter at what age. You should also write a *living will*. Should you suffer a terrible accident or debilitating disease, you want to leave your family and medical caregivers with directions on the kind of care you want.

def•i•ni•tion

A **living will** is an advance directive advising the medical community and your family what kind of care you want, should you be struck by a debilitating disease or accident.

Decide on how you want your remains taken care of. Do you want a traditional burial, or is cremation your choice? Perhaps you'd prefer a memorial service. Maybe you want everyone you love to get together, have a party, and tell funny stories about you. Think about it. Spell out your wishes.

Making Transitions

Change can be creative, momentous, frightening, revitalizing. It can open a new world of possibilities. There was a scene in the film classic *Gone with the Wind* when Scarlett, broke, with no resources other than her wit and daring, ripped down the old green velvet drapes from Tara's grand library and had Mammy transform them into a beautiful and fashionable dress. Look around you. The resources you need, resources that can be re-fabricated for other uses, are staring you in the face. Learn to recognize them.

The key to a mature future AQ consists of the ability to adapt to change, actively educating yourself throughout life, and preparing for the future. Balancing these three elements will enable you to maintain your perch on life's tight rope. It's healthy to believe that the golden age is ahead of you, rather than behind you. By living your life fully, as though you were going to live forever, you will surely have a ripe old future AQ.

The Least You Need to Know

- Ongoing education is essential to the well-lived life.
- Educational opportunities are everywhere.
- Maintaining a flexible mental attitude helps you adapt to change.
- Financial planning is key to ensuring a healthy future.
- Planning for the future is not the same as living in the future.

Part 4

The World Around You

Now you're going to step outside of yourself—outside your skin, outside your brain, outside your inner workings, and into the world around you: your family, your friends, your social life, your work and finances, and your community. Here you can be very content to come up with AQs right around your own age— or maybe a little bit more mature.

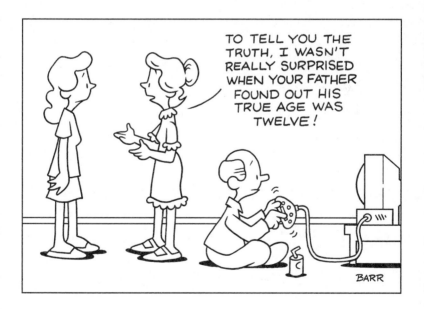

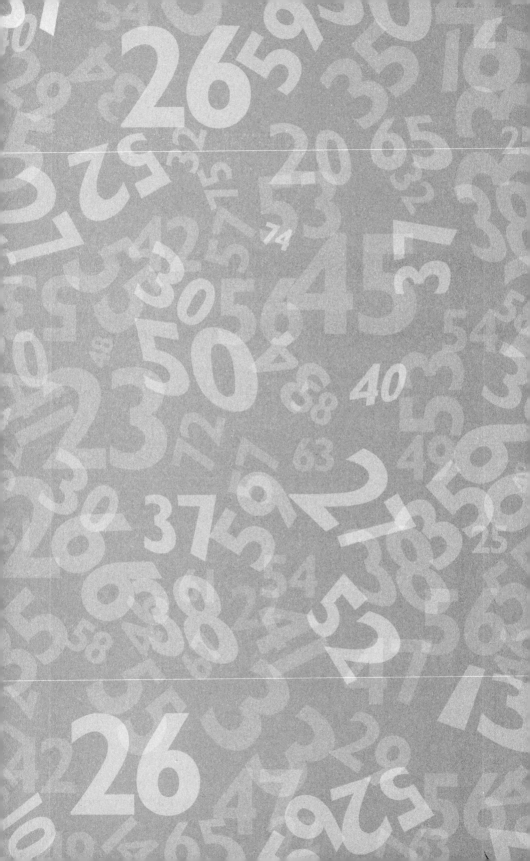

Chapter 10

Singleness True Age

In This Chapter

- ◆ Optimizing your singleness true age
- ◆ Benefits and challenges of the single life
- ◆ Single head-of-family households
- ◆ Differences of gender roles for singletons
- ◆ Rewards and difficulties of platonic friendships

Life's most enduring relationship is the one you have with yourself.

Whether or not you've chosen your independent state, you know, perhaps better than most, the many advantages and rewards to the single life. You can make major decisions without consensus; go where you like, when you feel like it; sleep when, where, and with whom you like; and have the satisfaction of knowing that you can take care of yourself all by yourself. If, that is, you are a mature singleton.

How to find out? Take the following quiz, of course!

Your Singleness True Age Quiz

1. What is your attitude toward being single?

    D. I enjoy it, but am open to having a partner.

    C. I'm unhappy about it.

    E. I like it and wish to remain so.

    F. I don't give it much thought.

2. Have you ever had intimate relationships of lasting value over a period of time?

    A. No, and I don't care to

    C. Once, but it didn't work out

    F. Yes, but my mate died

    D. Several

    B. No, and I'm sad about it

3. In which of the following circumstances do you live?

    D. Alone

    C. With platonic roommate(s)

    E. With dependent parent(s)

    D. With my young child/ren (under 25)

    B. With parent(s) upon whom I'm dependent

    H In assisted care, retirement community, etc.

    G. With my adult child/ren (over 25)

4. What is the state of your social life?

    C. I have platonic friends.

    A. I don't see people much; I'm a loner.

    D. I have a special friend whom I date exclusively.

    C. I date several friends.

    B. I'd like to be dating but I never meet anyone.

5. What is your attitude toward marriage?

   F. It's a fine institution for those able to handle it.

   B. In this day and age, what's the point?

   E. It's a very practical mode in our couples-focused society.

   C. If you want kids, fine; otherwise, why bother?

   A. Everyone should eventually marry.

6. What is the hardest part of being single for you?

   B. Spending evenings alone

   C. Lack of regular sex

   E. Not having children

   E. Being ostracized by our couples-focused society

   D. Having no one with whom to share decision-making and chores

   D. Having no one with whom to unburden myself or share special times

   F. Discrimination in business

7. Have you learned to take care of such annoying tasks as fixing a leaky faucet, changing the battery in your fire alarm, etc.?

   B. No; I always need help.

   F. Yes; I pride myself on being self-sufficient.

   D. Sometimes yes, sometimes no, depending on how complicated it is.

8. How much do you enjoy your own company?

   G. I'm perfectly content being by myself.

   F. I do enjoy my own company, but delight in the company of others, too.

   C. I don't like being alone much. I prefer having others around me.

9. If you live with roommates, what are your reasons for doing so?

    D. From the standpoint of finances, it is purely practical.

    B. I would be miserable living alone, with no one to talk to.

    E. I enjoy the camaraderie of companionship.

Scoring

Here's how to score your quiz:

1. Write in the letter for each answer in the "Letter" column.

2. Using the "Letter Values" list, find the value of points for each letter and write that number in the "Points" column.

3. Add up the points and write the total in the corresponding space.

4. Write in the *number of answers* you responded to for the section in the corresponding space and divide that number into the sum of points.

The result is your singleness true age!

Letter Values

A = 5 B = 15 C = 25 D = 35 E = 45 F = 55 G = 65 H = 75 I = 85 J = 95

Singleness True Age		
	Letter	**Points**
1.		
2.		
3.		
4.		
5.		
6.		
7.		
8.		
9.		
Total		
÷ #?s		
AQ		

Interpreting Your Score

Whether you're a Gen-X single or a senior citizen, you want your singleness AQ to be a mature one. If yours is in the 40s, you are probably quite independent, self-sufficient, and well-adjusted to being on your own. However, if your score is in the 20s or low 30s, it may be that you need to reassess your state of singledom. Go back and look at the questions to see where your answers were less mature than others. Similarly, if you end up in the 60s or higher, you, too, might benefit by reviewing the questions and your answers to see in which areas you are, perhaps, a bit inflexible.

It's necessary to bear in mind, too, that the experience of singledom is very different for different age groups. In your 20s and 30s, single life feels just fine for many and, in fact, may be a clear choice. You may not be interested in dating or marrying or even having a relationship. But once you hit middle age and have, perhaps, had a long-term relationship or two, the experience of singledom is often quite different. It is also different for those who live in a more urban setting than those who live in small towns or rural areas.

Whatever your age group or circumstances, chances are, if you had a mature self-image AQ, you're going to have a mature singleness AQ as well.

Living Alone

Some singles live with roommates, some live alone. There are advantages and disadvantages to both. When you live alone, you don't have to put up with your husband's employers or his dirty socks on the bathroom floor, your wife's in-laws or her panties hanging up to dry in the shower. You don't have to give away the cat because of your spouse's allergies, compromise your taste in furnishings, or desperately attempt to create some private space in your own home. You can live as simply or as lavishly as you choose (or can afford) without having to accommodate someone else's tastes, anxieties, or indulgences. You are free of the constant negotiations over even the smallest decision that exasperates so many married people. And if you want meatloaf three nights in a row, who's to stop you?

There are disadvantages to living alone, too. No one to review the day with when you get home from work. Nobody with whom to discuss the film you just watched. Yet the telephone and the Internet are there if you have the need to share. You also have to learn to be very self-sufficient, although that could be considered more of an advantage than a disadvantage. No one else is going to fix the stopped-up toilet at 3 in the morning; no one else is going to sew on your buttons, do your laundry, or apply a bandage to the finger you cut dicing potatoes for dinner. Actually, by living alone, you have great opportunities for learning skills, developing a strong identity, and gaining a deep awareness of your own needs and tastes. This is not to suggest that there aren't many special delights and lessons found in a solid marriage, but merely to affirm that singleness has its own special advantages and rewards.

Americans live in a couple's society that doesn't particularly embrace singledom; it's convinced that two is the only number. Unlike some cultures, where extended families and close-knit communities embrace their unmarried members, Western society is always trying to marry their singles off. This is true for all singletons, whether they're dyed-in-the-wool bachelors, widows, or divorcees.

How you respond to the question, posed to you for the umpteenth time, "How come you're not married?" is a challenge to your patience and your values. If yours is a defensive, "I want to be married, I just haven't met the right person," you will probably find you have a rather immature singleness AQ. The single life is not so much a choice as something you have to tolerate. But if you can respond with something like, "It's simply not part of my plan at this point in time," or, "I have many rewarding relationships without having to be married," you are likely one of those people who enjoys your single status and does very well by yourself, thank you very much. No doubt your AQ here will be a mature one.

One of the pitfalls for some singles is a tendency to socialize only with other singles by gravitating to singles bars, singles housing, singles parties, and singles clubs. While this separatism may be seen as attractive, it may cut you off from other segments of society, truncating potentially wonderful relationships with children and an older generation. The singleton whose social life is rich and varied, filled with married couples, children, and older people, as well as other singles, is going to be a far more satisfied individual than those who limit themselves to singles only.

Unless a conscious effort is made, social roles may also be more limited—no involvement with schools or scouts, unless, of course, you're raising children. Singles without children may see less of their parents and grandparents, too (although the opposite can be true—that is, singles may depend too much on their parents for their social life; this would decidedly lower their social AQ). Yet each of these limitations can be easily surmounted by simply becoming conscious of them and deciding to do something about it. Many singles, for example, broaden their interaction with other age groups by becoming a Big Brother or Sister, coaching at Little League games, taking friends' children for outings, or volunteering at a nursing home.

When it comes to the workplace, if you are single and don't have kids, it may be a positive factor. Assumptions may be made that you can spend long hours at work. In fact, at times, you may be taken advantage of and asked to do extra work since people think you don't have to rush home to make dinner or be with your family.

Building Relationships

Not all, but most, singles want to have a romantic relationship, even if they don't want to marry. The Internet abounds with dating services that try to match people up. Ironically, professionals in their 20s and 30s are finding "unprecedented difficulty in finding love in today's world," according to Jillian Straus, author of *Unhooked Generation*. After conducting 100 interviews in every major city in the States, this one-time producer of *The Oprah Winfrey Show* points out three major factors for why it's harder for today's young professionals to find a mate than it was a generation or two ago:

♦ There are so many more choices, it's harder to make one.

♦ In our multiple choice culture, there are so many opportunities to upgrade.

♦ The importance of relationships isn't as highly valued in corporate America as it once was.

Straus also talked about the myth that imbues one's thinking with the certainty that there is one person "out there" meant for you. That myth promulgates the idea that one will immediately recognize "the one" when they first meet, ignoring the real potential of relationships with those they meet along the way.

In our society, the author claims, people have developed an attitude of "Why suffer? Take Prozac." Why work at building a relationship when there are so many possible instant relationships out there? Straus advises those looking for love to cultivate patience; to avoid e-mail, text messaging, and IM; and to stop holding out for your "soul mate." Instead of looking to "upgrade," she suggests learning to work on the relationship you have. Sound advice from this 35-year-old who only recently married.

Many single people today enjoy an active sex life. For some, it's an ongoing relationship that has lasted a long time. Such couples have their own reasons for not living together. Nonetheless, they are a couple and will find the significant other AQ chapter as applicable to them as this one, if not more so.

For other singles, their sex lives consist of occasional or frequent brief encounters. While there may be great thrills to these liaisons, eventually they tend to wear thin. After a few years of it, one is usually not as eager to go through the by-then routine preliminaries of a sexual liaison; the relationship that does not deepen beyond a sexual one grows tired all too quickly.

There is also the concern today about sexually transmitted diseases. Not having a regular sexual partner, especially in the age of AIDS, means either having to do without or having to be very cautious, both quite stressful situations. If you're attracted to someone and want to have sex, how do you ask the questions or trust the answers if you don't really know that person?

Alternative Choices

Numerous singles have chosen abstinence over sexual involvement, some for religious reasons, some out of fear of STDs, some who simply do not enjoy sex, and some who simply want to wait until they find a mate. Whether or not you are sexually active or abstinent is immaterial to your singleness AQ. What does matter is how comfortable you are with the choices you've made.

Among certain subcultures, such as that of the male homosexual, a libertine lifestyle is more the custom rather than the exception. When AIDS came along in the 1980s, that changed drastically; but it seems to be making a comeback.

If you engage in a swinging lifestyle, juggling two or three affairs, or are a serial monogamist with a string of failed relationships behind you, will find that eventually it must come to an end if you are to develop any lasting and meaningful unions.

Wisdom of the Ages

You can only be young once. But you can always be immature.

—Dave Barry

Those singles who come up with a very young, perhaps even adolescent, sexuality AQ will quite likely have an immature singleness AQ as well.

Good Friends

Platonic friendships take on added importance for the singleton, frequently evolving into lifelong bonds that offer the support and nurturing everyone requires. A mature singleness AQ will invariably have a mature friendship AQ. Among some circles, lasting friendships may be difficult to maintain when the friend is of the opposite sex and is married. The married partner, particularly if he or she is not as close with the singleton, simply cannot handle the potential of sexual innuendo between their mate and the third party.

This may be more true among older singles. One woman, whose true age is 51, said, "I hate the fact that people are so narrow-minded that they think—most people still do—in couples. When a girlfriend has met a new man, suddenly we cannot meet all together, and I often get the comment that it would be so much easier if I had someone. It is not so much from male friends. I think my women friends are afraid of me being single; they claim that it is not so much fun for the man, to have two women to talk to during a dinner for example." Consequently, many close friendships are limited to members of one's own gender and couple status, with the not-infrequent exception of gay men and straight women. On the other hand, particularly in urban settings and among Gen-X singles, such a situation is simply not an issue. When it is an issue, rather than risk the loss of a good and true friend, all parties should sit down and have a good talk, relieving tensions and possible misunderstandings.

Men have the excellent advantage of buddy systems such as the Elks, the Masons, and professional and veterans' associations which bring men together who have common ground. On a less formal basis, buddies watch TV sports and play sports. The relationships they form can be strong, but they are usually of a quite different texture than the intimate friendships women often form. Perhaps that's because men are not encouraged to be open and confessional with one another. Rewarding as these friendships may be, the lack of intimacy for the single man can generate a strong feeling of loneliness.

When friends get married, or if you have recently divorced, you may find married friends distancing themselves from you. They may simply be more occupied with nesting and raising a family then they were before, or, if you're newly single, you may have more time on your hands than you did before.

Wisdom of the Ages _____

"So yeah, anyway—I'm thirty-four and my mother is desperate for
me to get married. She thinks settling down is what you should be
doing at thirty-four. How would she like it if I turned to her the day
she hits eighty and said: 'Hey, Mum—when are you going to break your
hip? All your friends are breaking theirs'?"

—Sue Margolis, *Spin Cycle*, 2001

Let friends know how thrilled you are about their marriage or new
baby. Offer to baby-sit or help paint the living room. Make it clear from
the outset that you are paying your own tab when you go out to eat. If
you handle such social situations forthrightly and with confidence and
assurance, you will no doubt be quite successful at maintaining and
deepening your friendships with couples as well as other singles.

There's one special problem facing single women in midlife who never
have borne a child: they must face up to shutting off that possibility, a
reality men do not have to deal with. Of course, for some women, that
has been a choice. But for many it is not. More and more women in this
position are opting for adoption or, using a sperm donor bank, in-vitro
fertilization.

Single Parenthood

A growing phenomenon, single parenthood brings with it its own challenges and rewards. In 1977, there were 9.2 million one-parent homes
in the United States; in 2004 there were 19.5 million. While most one-
parent homes are headed by either divorced or abandoned women, some
are headed by men, some by women who have chosen to adopt or bear
a child but not to marry, and some by homosexual parents, especially
lesbians.

A single person with children has some very special needs. Housing in
an environment compatible for both your offspring and your social life;
privacy and discretion in sexual encounters when a child is in the home;
dealing with well-meaning but snoopy neighbors, teachers, etc.; and
juggling all the demands of parenthood and work without a partner.

How Many Candles?

A marketing consultant in Silicon Valley, this never-married singleton lives a comfortable life in her own home. Very conscious of nutrition and health, she has a medical AQ of 25 and a physical fitness AQ of 19. Despite living far away from other family members, she gets together with them whenever she can. She's close with some of her three siblings, but not all of them. Raised in a home where there was verbal and physical affection, her family AQ is 50. She enjoys her single state, though she'd be open to the right partner. The only real problem she has with it is the lack of someone to share special times, decision-making, and such (singleness AQ 35). Her social life makes up for a lot of that, however, as she enjoys a very satisfying circle of friends with whom she goes to events with. She's very active with a local club, and goes to meetings weekly (community AQ 51). Her true age is 46. Her chronological age: 59. This professional is leading a rich, rewarding single

When income is limited to one paycheck (42 percent of all households have two income earners), money can become another challenging issue. While many responsible divorced fathers help support their children and assist in tending to their needs, taking them on vacations and covering other expenses, too many ignore these obligations, often compelling ex-wives with children to find public or private assistance.

Single people with children may find themselves discriminated against in employment practices, even though it is a violation of their civil rights. An employer may be concerned that you need to take time off when the kids are sick or leave early to pick them up from school. While it is true that, as middle age approaches, the chance of finding a new mate decreases, particularly for women, and even more so for women with children, for many unmarried people, children are a strong motivation for carrying on and leading a productive life.

One 55-year-old woman, divorced in the foreign country where she and her ex-husband had lived 30 years earlier, said of her return to the States, "I came back to this country with 45 pounds of personal possessions, my marriage destroyed, and two little people. Many of my friends in their 40s were having nervous breakdowns, and I thought, 'Heavens, that's a marvelous thing to do. When you have a nervous breakdown, somebody else has to take over everything. My situation is made for a nervous breakdown.' But I didn't seem to be made for one. I looked at my little people, and I knew there was no way—the monetary end of it never occurred to me. I just knew I'd take care of them."

Widowhood

The suffering of widowhood is an agonizing and desolate circumstance. The death of one's soul mate is one of the major crises of life. It presents serious problems of personal adjustment and mental health: widowed people typically have higher death rates, a greater incidence of mental disorders, and a higher suicide rate than their married counterparts. There were more than 13.5 million widows in 2004.

Friends may be at a loss as to how to deal with the recently widowed person. Her despair and preoccupation with death may be uncomfortable for others, especially in this society where death tends to be a hush-hush subject.

Sometimes people shun mourners out of discomfort and fear. In-laws, no longer bound by blood, may distance themselves from their widowed brother- or sister-in-law. New friends, always hard to come by, may seem impossible to cultivate during this needy time of sorrow. Most newly widowed persons would have a low singleness AQ. But for the most part, good friends and family form a safety net for loved ones in need.

It's important that the newly widowed take time out to grieve properly for their lost mates. Only when the cycle of grief, in all its stages, has been worked through, can the bereaved detach themselves from past bonds and be ready to choose and enjoy a new life.

Clearly, the more dependent a man or woman has been on his or her spouse, whether for identity or economic support, the more difficult will be the period

Birthday Blahs

If you are newly widowed, take care not to rush into any big changes, like moving to a new city, or even dating. It is always optimal to remain in your same dwelling for the first year. Fight the tendency to give away clothes and possessions: once done, it cannot be undone. Store things for a while. Take your time.

of readjustment after the loss of a mate, whether by divorce or death. Those who have alternate interests and a variety of roles will find adjustment to being alone less taxing. There are many self-help groups to enable the newly bereaved or divorced to learn to understand their experiences, discover options open to them, and work though the stages of grief, which psychologists have identified as the following:

♦ Denial: "This can't be happening to me."

♦ Anger: "Why is this happening? Who is to blame?"

♦ Bargaining: "Make this not happen, and in return I will …."

♦ Depression: "I'm too sad to do anything."

♦ Acceptance: "I'm at peace with what has happened."

It generally takes about two years to work through these stages. Mind you, they are not necessarily sequential; you can start in the middle, go back and forth, get stuck in one area, or skip another altogether. The order of things is unique to each individual. But if you do find yourself unable to work through your grief in the customary amount of time, it might be advisable to seek professional help.

In her tender book *Widow*, Lynn Caine wrote, "I am convinced that if I had known the facts of grief before I had to experience them, it would not have made my grief less intense …. But it would've allowed me to hope. It would have given me courage. I would have known that once my grief was worked through, I would be joyful again."

Hope, sometimes, is all we have to hold our lives together. Hope can be offered to those in mourning by sharing their burdens and fears, as well as helping them see the future in less bleak terms. Such sharing will speed the mending process, enabling the griever to mature and achieve a singleness AQ compatible with his or her own age group.

Someone to Share With

Not all single people live alone, of course. Many live with other family members or friends (we do not refer here to cohabitants, but to platonic relationships). Such unions can be very effective in relieving stress, both economically (where two paychecks ease household bills) and socially. Having someone with whom to review the day's activities, to dine with, to help care for and be cared for by, and to share decision-making, does much to create emotional stability. Such people would be candidates for mature singleness AQs.

How Many Candles?

Born in Singapore and living in the Muang District of Thailand, this gal is somewhat underweight and has low blood pressure. Still, she can take four to five flights of stairs without difficulty, is fairly flexible, despite not participating in any regular exercise or sports (physical fitness AQ 35), and in decent medical condition (medical AQ 32). She doesn't do much in the way of brain anaerobics, but she reads a great deal, and does physical aerobics at least three times a week. Getting out in nature isn't her strong suit, but she writes every day (brain AQ 42). While she enjoys sex, she has been almost entirely inactive (sexuality AQ 51) and has no-one special in her life (singleness AQ 30). Deciding to go back to school, this student lives with her parents, upon whom she's dependent—and very close (family AQ 49). Her true age is 46. Her chronological age: 30. If she developed more of a social life, she would not have to be so dependent on her parents and would give her-self more opportunities to meet someone special. And if she quit smoking and started exercising, her true age would be more in accord with her chronological age.

There is a very special place that a pet can have in the life of a single person. A pet is someone to come home to; someone to cuddle with; someone other than yourself to be responsible for. As one single put, "I get so much joy from having my two kitties in my life. My cats are 'my kids.'" Having a pet has been proven to be therapeutic for shut-ins and the elderly. There is little question that, like any healthy companionate relationship, it will raise your singleness AQ.

The single life holds many joys, many rewards, and many challenges. There is no better or worse, no right or wrong, to one's social status—married, divorced, widowed, never married, cohabiting, single, straight, or gay. Everyone, after all, is after the same thing: a rich and meaning-ful life filled with friendship and challenges, comfort and health.

The Least You Need to Know

- The single life can be richly rewarding.

- Single parents face particularly difficult circumstances.

- Singles who want a lasting love relationship need to focus on building rather than shopping for one.

- Single women generally have more challenges than do single men.

- Friendships fill many gaps in the single life.

- Newly divorced or widowed people need to take time to grieve before embarking on their new lives as singletons.

Chapter 11

Significant Other True Age

In This Chapter

- Optimizing your significant other age quotient
- Creating a lasting relationship
- Reaping the benefits of marriage
- Surviving middle age
- Weathering changing relationships

How old is your relationship? Mind you, that's not the same question as "How many years have you been together?" There are unions of 25 or 40 years' duration that may, on the AQ scale, turn out to be quite young—which is to say, immature. Other, shorter-lived coupleships may be so evolved as to rate a very high AQ. Your significant other AQ depends not upon the length of your union, but upon its depth and dimension. This chapter examines (or rediscovers) the pivot upon which a mature relationship revolves.

Your Significant Other True Age Quiz

Because of the similarities among marrieds and cohabitants in terms of mutual needs and satisfactions, the legal status of your partnership has no bearing whatsoever on your significant other AQ.

1. How is your relationship with your mate?

   F. Highly satisfactory

   E. Somewhat satisfactory

   B. Very unsatisfactory

   D. Sometimes it's good, sometimes it's bad

2. Are you having, or have you had, extramarital relationships?

   E. Never

   D. Once

   C. Two or three times

   B. Four or more times

3. Do you and your partner share recreational activities (bowling, hiking, playing cards, dancing, etc.)?

   J. Never

   H. Once or twice a year

   F. Several times a year

   E. At least once a month

   D. Weekly

   C. Daily

4. What is your level of interdependence?

   C. My mate is too dependent on me.

   B. I am too dependent on my mate.

   A. We are too dependent on each other.

   E. Our interdependence is well balanced.

   C. We are too independent of each other.

5. Do you and your mate share decision-making?

    E. When it's important

    D. Only if it's convenient

    A. Never or hardly ever

    C. Almost always

6. Do you and your mate share private time together?

    E. Yes, on a regular basis

    D. Whenever we can squeeze it in

    C. Occasionally

    B. Very infrequently

    A. Never or hardly ever

7. How has the passage of time affected your relationship?

    H. It hasn't been affected much.

    D. It has vastly improved.

    A. It has deteriorated.

    E. It has acquired a more even keel.

8. In a marriage where both partners work, how should housework be handled?

    B. The woman should do it all.

    F. Assuming fairness, each should do what he or she is best suited for.

    E. If affordable, they should hire a housekeeper.

    D. It should be evenly divided.

9. If you were faced with divorce, which statement would best apply to you?

    C. If my partner asked, I'd grant it.

    D. If I were chronically unhappy, I'd ask for it.

    A. I'd never divorce, no matter what.

    B. If I were chronically unhappy, I'd try to learn to live with it.

    E. I'd try anything to save the marriage first.

10. If your mate is going through a hard time (e.g., illness, loss of parent, inheritance, sibling rivalry), some difficulty not shared by you, what is your usual response?

    F. I'm sympathetic but won't interfere.

    H. I'm sympathetic and try to find solutions.

    J. I'm sympathetic, but only offer help if asked.

    B. I feel annoyed and alienated.

    E. I feel helpless and frustrated.

    A. I wish the problem would just go away so things could be normal again.

Scoring

Here's how to score your quiz:

1. Write in the letter for each answer in the "Letter" column.

2. Using the "Letter Values" list, find the value of points for each letter and write that number in the "Points" column.

3. Add up the points and write the total in the corresponding space.

4. Write in the *number of answers* you responded to for the section in the corresponding space and divide that number into the sum of points.

The result is your significant other true age!

Letter Values

A = 5 B = 15 C = 25 D = 35 E = 45 F = 55 G = 65 H = 75 I = 85 J = 95

Significant Other True Age		
	Letter	**Points**
1.		
2.		
3.		
4.		
5.		
6.		
7.		
8.		
9.		
10.		
Total		
÷ #?s		
AQ		

Interpreting Your Score

If you've been married 30 years and come out with an AQ of 25, you probably have some serious work to do on strengthening the bonds of your partnership. If you've been together only 5 or 10 years and have an AQ of 40, you are batting a thousand! When it comes to your significant other AQ, a result somewhere between 38ish and 52ish is where you want to be, as it signifies a relationship that is flourishing, mature, and resilient.

Love

The thrill of love! Poets write of it. Heroes die for it. What other emotion is so purely ecstatic, so utterly delicious? When you feel the tremendous power of attraction that is the beginning of love, when you acknowledge that the two of you "have chemistry," you're more on target than you might have thought.

Scientists, in rooting out the reasons why love feels so good, have discovered that when you're attracted to someone, the brain creates dopamine, a chemical that gives you a natural high. Then serotonin, another feel-good chemical, kicks in.

You actually begin to learn how to love when you're just a baby. You quickly learned that a smile brings tenderness, caring, affection. As you grew into toddler-hood, you became very affectionate with your parents, your siblings, your friends, freely dispensing hugs and kisses. The lessons continued right through adolescence, when the focus on sex and, most commonly, the opposite sex, came into play. Dopamine has a field day with puppy love. When people say they're "addicted to love," they're not kidding. Dopamine is the same stuff that keeps drug addicts addicted; it is also the stuff that keeps lovers addicted to each other.

Once the thrill of new love is past and the "I do's" have been said, the journey of a long-term relationship begins. Someone still has to do the dishes, take out the trash, walk the dog, and change the baby's diapers. "Companionate love," psychologists call it. That's when the brain starts putting out more of two other chemicals—oxytocin and vasopressin. Pregnant women and nursing mothers are flooded with oxytocin—and so are their live-in mates. These are bonding chemicals that keep people, especially parents, attached like Velcro to the objects of their love.

Freud's original *Project for Scientific Psychology*—abandoned in 1893—attempted to relate all psychological events to cellular biology and chemistry. It's beginning to look like that is fundamentally true. But while scientists parse out the chemical cocktail that makes people fall in love, stay in love, or fall out of love, you are still left to make the most of your relationships.

Actress Shelley Winters once said, "It was so cold out, I almost got married." A flimsy reason, you say? At least it's practical. Falling in love is wonderful; it's exhilarating. But taking an oath to live your life with someone based only on romantic love and good sex may be an even flimsier reason to wed than the desire to stay warm. The expectations of romantic love are extravagant.

Marriage and Other Long-Term Relationships

Marriage offers many legal benefits, ranging from property and inheritance rights to legal guardianship of children to retirement benefits. But whether you're bound legally or not, studies show that fidelity is just as important among cohabitants as it is among marrieds, and that the division of household labor is just as traditional, with the woman bearing the brunt of the labor. Cohabitants are confronted with much of the same problems as their married counterparts, with one additional conundrum: whether or not to marry.

In the gay and lesbian world, cohabitation is usually the only option available, although many countries and some states now allow for civil unions, which grant same-sex partners certain legal rights that they otherwise would not have.

Wisdom of the Ages

At every party there are two kinds of people— those who want to go home and those who don't. The trouble is, they are usually married to each other.

—Ann Landers

Though there are times when long-term relationships may feel dull and routine, they are, for the most part, good for you. Research shows that married people live longer and are healthier than unmarried people. Perhaps it is because the stresses of life are relieved somewhat when one has a partner with whom to share them. Cardiovascular disease, cancer, respiratory diseases, even mental illness, all have lower rates among marrieds, and even more so for men. (Married men do tend to be about 20 percent more overweight than their single buddies, however.) There are, of course, instances where relationships do more harm than good, which is dealt with later on in the chapter.

Mates tend to watch out for each other. A wife will remind her husband he needs his annual physical checkup. "Women are really the mental- and physical-health housekeepers for a marriage," hypothesizes psychologist Janice Kiecolt-Glaser of Ohio State University. Men are important caretakers of the home, too—and the safety of their family: they'll remember to change the furnace filter, clean out the gutters, seal the windows. Unless you've got a whole lot of money, how else can you enjoy a full-time companion-caretaker? Marriage is healthy, and a natural offshoot of love.

But how do you know if you're making a good choice? Despite a minimum of 12 years of education, few people learn any of the practicalities of couple dynamics. Most of you have good common sense. You try to be pragmatic in your decision-making. Yet practicalities are rarely cited as reasons for marriage. Most people marry or live together because they fall in love. But unless they're very lucky, couples who marry strictly for romantic love may find themselves among the spiraling numbers of divorces in this country.

Birthday Blahs

The dream of rescue that leads to many marriages—he will fulfill me, she will make my life complete—can be very unrealistic. Such exaggerated expectations in what a partner will provide more often than not lead to disappointment, despair, and divorce.

So you "fall" in love and marry. After a few years, you may notice something is amiss in your marital bliss. You awaken from your dream of rescue to find yourself in a nightmare of misguided hopes and unfulfilled desires. By now you're in your 30s or 40s. There are children to consider, and ties and obligations to an extended family and the community.

Tender Loving Care

Whatever it is that impels people to fall in love, certain things need to happen if the bond is going to hold:

- ◆ Idealization (she's the most beautiful, the most clever; he's the sexiest, the brightest)—While the realities of daily living may tone down one's initial impressions, a modicum must remain if the relationship is to have a chance for survival.

- ◆ Trust—Though it rarely comes all at once, the seeds must be there from the get-go, and it must continue to grow. When trust breaks down, the relationship crumbles.

- Identification (when he's frustrated, you're frustrated; when she's in pain, you can't bear it)—An offshoot of intimacy, it flowers into understanding and empathy of one another's needs and sensitivities.

- Complementary—Each mate makes essential and distinct contributions to the relationship.

One of the things to look out for is dependency. Many have the illusion that their partners ought to "complete" them: if you're shy, he'll make friends for you; if you're insecure, he'll be brave for you; if you cannot perform basic household chores, she'll handle it for both of you. While interdependence is a part of any healthy relationship, too much dependency can breed resentment. Work to expand your activities outside the home and the workplace: join a hiking group, a bridge club, a service organization.

There are many ingredients that go into a mature and fulfilling relationship, including compassion, compatibility, respect, and thoughtfulness. And liking. It's important to continue *liking* each other, to be friends. It's imperative to work at the rela-

Wisdom of the Ages

I have yet to hear a man ask for advice on how to combine marriage and a career.

—Gloria Steinem

tionship, consistently reinforcing it: it is a living thing! Think of your mate as a true partner—just as you might in a business relationship: appreciate and encourage her contributions and strengths.

Here are the tools, the *sine qua non*, of making a long-term relationship work. All of them are in your control:

- Constant inquiry: Check in with your mate. How is she feeling? Did he sleep well? What's happening at work?

- Disclosure: Deep concerns and hurts must be revealed, even though it can be very painful.

- Consideration: Don't just barge ahead with plans without consulting each other.

- Appreciation: Be very specific. "Thank you for doing the shopping today," "I couldn't have filled in that job application without your input," etc. Little things do mean a lot.

◆ Open admiration: Again, be specific: "What a great meal that was," "You have such patience with the kids," "I'm so impressed with your thoroughness in handling our finances," etc.

◆ Positive reinforcement: "You can finish that 10K—I know you can," "If you want to go back to school, we'll find a way," etc.

◆ Affection: Morning hugs. Holding hands. Saying "I love you" every single day!

How Many Candles?

Both husband and wife work, but aren't thrilled with their careers, which afford them only a modest income (his financial AQ is 30; hers is 42). It's a second marriage for him, a first for her. They have two children and a good family relationship, although the man is not so close with his parents or siblings (her family AQ is 42; his is 36). Very sexually compatible (his sexuality AQ is 25; hers is 21), they have a good relationship, though he feels he's a little too dependent on her (his significant other AQ is 35; hers is 44). She seems more fulfilled with their social life than he (her social AQ is 48; his is 36). His true age is 45; hers is 51. They've been married 13 years. His chronological age is 50; hers is 44. While they both have a rather immature sexuality AQ, it seems to work for them. But she seems more mature and content with her life than her husband does. He needs to find ways to improve his social life and to lessen his dependence on his wife.

In a good relationship, all these elements continue to deepen as time goes by. A solidly united middle-aged couple is more trusting, more identified, and more attached than they were as young lovers.

Sex, Money, and Relationships

Even though you explored your sexuality AQ in Chapter 5, it's wise to at least briefly review the subject in terms of the dynamics of your relationship. Same goes for money, which will be dealt with more thoroughly in Chapter 14.

In long-term relationships, sex can get into a repetitious rut. When children are on the scene and enter adolescence, an atmosphere of self-consciousness may further reduce sexual activities. More strain on sexual relations may arrive during the transitional years of your 40s and 50s: the kids have grown up and are moving out; your grandparents are dying; your parents are moving to retirement or nursing homes; advancement at work may demand more responsibilities and more time, or you may find yourself at a dead end.

Exhaustion, frustration, an empty nest—a decreased sexual drive is not infrequently the result. A common reaction to that upsetting experience is to blame one's spouse. Perhaps it isn't coincidental that divorce rates begin to spiral in the 40 to 50 age range.

How Many Candles?

This couple never fails to celebrate birthdays, anniversaries, and Valentine's Day with a romantic evening out. They cook and dine together daily. They share many interests and spend a great deal of their leisure time together. They both work at home and have partnered on several business projects. They often disagree on cultural matters (his social AQ is 46; hers is 45), but are akin on spiritual ones (his spiritual AQ is 65; hers is 82). Not a day goes by without hugs, kisses, and "I love you." His significant other AQ is 43 and hers is 42. His true age is 55 and hers is 53. His chronological age is 58; hers is 66. They've been together 34 years. This couple has managed to keep their relationship lively; they stay attuned to one another due to a mature approach to society and each other.

Panic about sexual prowess will sometimes plunge one headlong into an adulterous affair. It seems the "seven-year itch" is more likely to be the 15- or 20-year itch. But infidelity need not bring about the dissolution of a marriage: there are many ways it can be dealt with—starting with candor, then moving on to forgiveness and acceptance, and finally a renewed promise of faithfulness. But the carnage of jealousy can mangle the best of marriages. And it is jealousy, not the act of adultery, that is the most destructive.

Then there's money, a symbol of power in many unions. The way it is handled is indicative of the personalities and levels of maturity involved. When money becomes an issue, it is rarely the amount that is the problem (with the exception of poverty), but how the money is being used—to control, punish, or manipulate.

The changing roles for men and women in Western society has had an even more tumultuous part in creating ego-strife and power plays between husband and wife. Though men earn 30 percent higher wages than do women in the same jobs, a woman's earning power may still be a threat to the traditional male ego—another arrow in the quiver of middle-aged divorce.

Life is messy. Maturity involves acknowledging confusion and not having all the answers. It means confessing to feelings of helplessness and futility. Mature individuals have the guts to admit vulnerability. If you play the game of all-knowing father or supermom to your children and your mate, you stunt those relationships as surely as you stunt your own growth.

So often barriers are created by freezing the image you had of your partner at the time of the inception of the relationship. That is as immature and unfair as letting yourself become stuck in a time warp of your younger years. You can no more expect your partner to remain the same than you can expect yourself to.

Divorce

Every relationship has its ups and downs, on a daily, monthly, even a yearly basis. It's the way those ups and downs are handled that dictates the maturity or immaturity of the partners involved. It's essential to allow yourself to step back and take a look at the overall picture of those hills and valleys and be able to decide when there are just too many low points for the relationship to continue.

Actually, most divorces occur after a very brief period of time—under two years. Marriages of long duration—10, 20, even 30 years—are the ones most difficult to dissolve. Long-term relationships usually involve child custody, property rights, and all sorts of painful and messy decisions. But more than that is the pain of separating the thousands of threads that have created the tapestry of a life together.

Separation not only means starting over again, it also usually means doing so alone. The longer you've been married, the older you are and the stranger is the experience of starting off on your own, perhaps for the first time, if you married very young. You may be so frightened of feeling isolated, lonely, and vulnerable that the inevitability of divorce is postponed for years. Misery with the familiar, it seems, is often preferable to the unknown.

The question as to whether or not a marriage should be clung to can only be answered by the people involved. But it should be noted that, friendly advice to the contrary, most unhappy marriages do severe psychic damage to the men and women brutalized by their own and each other's resentments.

Wisdom of the Ages

My wife Mary and I have been married for forty-seven years and not once have we had an argument serious enough to consider divorce; murder, yes, but divorce, never.

—Jack Benny

Everyone, of course, makes mistakes—and marriage is sometimes one of them. Forgiving oneself for such an error is as supreme an act as forgiving another. When divorce is inevitable, view it as a chapter in your life in which difficult lessons were learned, lessons that can lead to a richer future. Divorce needn't be looked upon as defeat. A good divorce should be as much celebrated as a good marriage.

Your significant other AQ can be kept mature and healthy by learning to anticipate certain inevitable changes—in yourself and in your partner. It is vital to be prepared for such changes, and be willing to make accommodations, eager for new adventures in a state of readiness and maturity, hand in hand with your mate. In such a way, you can strive for a significant other AQ at least on par with your chronological age—although preferably "older."

The Least You Need to Know

- The benefits of a healthy relationship are far ranging.

- A solid marriage is held together by specific, essential ingredients.

- Middle age is the riskiest period in a relationship.

- Divorce can be the best option and a positive move.

- If relationships don't grow and change with time, they can get in a rut.

Chapter 12

Family True Age

In This Chapter

- Optimizing your family age quotient
- Creating strong families
- Relating to parents as an adult child
- Encouraging independence in children—and in oneself
- Adjusting to changing family composition

Whether or not we would have chosen the family we were born into, we're usually stuck with them. It makes sense to make the best of it. And the best can be very good indeed. A "good family" is an invaluable asset not only while we're growing up, but when we strike out on our own as well.

The varying levels of maturity within the family unit—parent to child, child to parent, and siblings to one another, and the way in which the family unit relates to society—are the ingredients upon which the family AQ is based.

Your Family True Age Quiz

When considering your answers to the family true age quiz, feel free to include stepparents or guardians in your assessment. If you have no children of your own but there are children who have been central to your life—nieces and nephews or a ward—feel free to consider them in your answers.

1. What was the atmosphere of your home when you were growing up?

    J. Loving and supportive

    H. Supportive and loving, but critical

    E. Demanding, loving, and critical

    B. Critical and punitive

    A. Physically abusive and alienating

    C. Left to my own devices most of the time

    D. Loving, but not tuned in to me

2. If your parent(s) are still living, how much time and attention do you devote to them?

    A. More than I'd like

    C. Not as much as I'd like

    E. Enough to make everyone happy

    B. Not at all

3. What is/was the level of love and affection demonstrated in your family?

    J. Lots, physical and verbal

    H. Some, physical and verbal

    F. Verbal only; a fair amount

    E. Physical only; a fair amount

    B. Very little of either

    A. None

4. In general, what is your current relationship with your sibling(s)?

    G. Very close

    F. Somewhat close

    C. Somewhat alienated

    B. Very alienated

    E. Close with some, not with others

5. How has your relationship with your child/ren altered over the years?

    D. Gotten closer

    C. Drifted apart

    E. Always been good; still is

    B. Always been lousy; still is

6. What is your current relationship with your children?

    F. Very close

    E. Somewhat close

    C. Somewhat alienated

    B. Very alienated

7. How do you feel about your relationship with your child/ren?

    B. Somewhat discontented

    H. Very contented

    A. Very discontented

    F. Somewhat contented

    C. Don't have much of one

8. How much of your social life is comprised of family gatherings and functions?

    C. All of it

    F. Frequently

    D. Only for special occasions

    E. Get together whenever we can, regardless of distance

    B. None of it

9. If your child/ren have grown and left home, how do you feel about it?

   F. Freer

   A. Abandoned

   C. Useless

   B. Alone

   J. Glad for them

   D. Relieved for myself

10. If your adult child/ren still live at home, how do you feel?

    C. Can't wait for them to get out of the house

    E. Pleased to have them as long as they do their share

    B. Wish they'd stay forever

    D. Feel frustrated for them

11. If you do not have children, how do you feel about it?

    C. Unhappy, but never could have any and won't adopt

    H. It is my choice, a good one for me

    B. Never gave it much thought

    E. Plan on having some later

    H. Disappointed, but fully accepting

12. Does your household family eat meals together?

    F. At least once a day

    E. At least three to five times weekly

    C. Only on weekends

    B. Rarely

Scoring

Here's how to score your quiz:

1. Write in the letter for each answer in the "Letter" column.

2. Using the "Letter Values" list, find the value of points for each letter and write that number in the "Points" column.

3. Add up the points and write the total in the corresponding space.

4. Write in the *number of answers* you responded to for the section in the corresponding space and divide that number into the sum of points.

The result is your family true age!

Letter Values

A = 5 B = 15 C = 25 D = 35 E = 45 F = 55 G = 65 H = 75 I = 85 J = 95

Family True Age		
	Letter	**Points**
1.		
2.		
3.		
4.		
5.		
6.		
7.		
8.		
9.		
10.		
11.		
12.		
Total		
÷ #?s		
AQ		

Interpreting Your Score

As with all "The World Around You" categories, what you want to aim for here is a mature AQ, somewhere between 38 and 52. If you find yours is much lower than 38, it would be wise to look over the questions to discover where you may lack maturity in your family relationships. On the other hand, if you have an AQ over 60, the quiz may indicate areas to you where you are, perhaps, too dependent, or not expressive in your relations.

For example, one 33-year-old single had a solid family AQ of 43; not only were her family relationships very close, but they had improved over the years; whereas a 43-year-old doctor, married with children, had a family AQ of 63; his significant other AQ was 35. He was not happy in his marriage and did not have a close relationship with his wife, his children, or his parents!

The Family Unit

At their most basic level, families provide food, clothing, shelter, and health care for their members. But these same provisions could come from an institution. What makes each family special and unique is the provision of emotional bonding: family is one of the few places where love and companionship is offered without asking anything in return. That is its bedrock.

Family is the procreating tool for humankind and the basic socializing tool of civilization. It is the core of the social and economic life of the community and the spearhead of spiritual life.

Children swiftly accustom themselves to their roles as underlings to their parents, and peer, rival, or master of their siblings. But these roles change and shift in adulthood:

- Adult child to—and later caretaker for—your parents.

- Parent to growing or grown children; later still, grandparent.

- Peer to siblings who may once have been your rivals, your masters, or your slaves.

So there you are—stuck in the middle, neither fish nor fowl. These three major relationships are what will establish your family AQ.

Each family must have a breadwinner and a homemaker. At one time these were distinct roles, the former usually being the man's role and the latter the woman's. But today, more often than not, these functions overlap: 42 percent of all households have two income earners. And both male earners today also tend to household and child-rearing tasks (some more, some less). When children arrive, both parents serve as models to the growing child, ideally demonstrating hospitality, self-sufficiency, honesty, conscientiousness, fairness, and affection.

Affection is the glue that holds a family together. Without it, family members become detached and break away from the central core. Affection helps relieve the pressure and duress that are natural components of living and working together. Like the cream that rises to the top of whole raw milk, it isn't the most vital part, but it is the richest.

Family provides a place to share, celebrate, recuperate, and commiserate.

Parent to Your Children, Child to Your Parent

As you strike out on your own and start your own family, you'll most likely find that you cannot abandon the ties that bind you to your parents and siblings. Parents and siblings have a marked impact on your life, as may grandparents, aunts, uncles, and cousins with whom you've been close. Yet the dynamics of these relationships change. It's a complicated adjustment, one that can take years.

It is a tremendous transition to go from being an independent adult with few responsibilities to being a parent. In addition to grappling with the myriad demands and adjustments of parenthood, there may be a marked transition in the relationship with your own parents. If you took the family AQ quiz six months before becoming a parent and again six months later, you would see a big difference in your AQ.

If your parents—and your grandparents—attempt to take on their old role of parent with your children, you're going to find yourself at odds with them. Such conflicts can put a real strain on your relationship with your parents. How can this be avoided?

Prevention is the smartest move. Before the baby comes, you and your spouse could sit down with your parents and let them know you've thought seriously

Wisdom of the Ages

Familiarity breeds contempt—and children.

—Mark Twain

about how you want to raise your children. Tell them you learned a great deal from them and intend on using many of those lessons. But you've also come up with some ideas of your own that you intend to put into practice. Ask for their cooperation at the outset.

Such a conversation can occur anywhere along the continuum of child-rearing, of course, and may have to occur several times. The important thing is to keep the door open: you want your children to have an opportunity to have a marvelous relationship with their grandparents. This will enable a mature family AQ for all of you!

Grandparents must come to learn to keep their philosophies on child-rearing to themselves and allow their adult children to do the work of parenting. They may feel that, on some level, they are being displaced. But if they can refrain from meddling, and simply observe; if they can acknowledge that their children are fully entitled to do things very differently than they did, the likelihood of being included and valued increases.

Optimize Your AQ

Opinions about how your children are raising their children can be shared with friends, but if you older parents want to maintain a good relationship with your adult children, it would be wise to refrain from sharing those opinions with them.

The new parents may still be struggling to separate out from being their parents' child and may feel guilty, resentful, or insecure about their new status as a parent. But it's vital for the new parents to set their own parameters for their family. Find a balance between respecting your parents and holding firm to the fact that this is your time to establish your own customs and routines. Try to include parents and grandparents as often as possible, but with the understanding they must adapt to your ways. Let them know they're still important to you—and to your children.

More than 80 percent of older people live within an hour's drive from at least one of their grown children. This proximity can benefit both parties by making it possible for family members to care for one another during illness, baby-sit younger children, help out with house and repairs, celebrate birthdays and other holidays together, and all in all have deeper relationships.

These are all bonding activities that enrich the lives of families.

How Many Candles?

A mother of three young children living in New Orleans, this gal has worked as a high-powered partnership-development consultant. Brought up Catholic in a small rural town, she no longer considers herself religious, though she still goes to church once or twice a month. She hasn't found her spiritual path yet, but feels deeply spiritual (spiritual AQ 71). Juggling motherhood and work has not been particularly satisfying to her, but household finances are solid enough (financial AQ 46). She has a strong self-image (self-image AQ 73), a good social life (social AQ 52), and close family ties (family AQ 55), including a positive, solid relationship with her husband (significant other AQ 45). Her true age is 58. Her chronological age: 42. As her children grow and gain some independence, she won't feel quite so strapped down by them, which will lower her family AQ a bit. She also will have more time for her social circle, which will also equalize her social AQ a bit. The mature true age, however, is really a result of the good work she does for herself and her spiritual life.

When older parents and their adult children find their way toward a healthy mutuality, they will achieve a mature family AQ, for that is based on psychological security, affection, and mutuality with both one's parents, siblings, and, of course, significant other and offspring.

Parenting

It isn't easy to tell the truth, especially when it might cause your child's lower lip to tremble and tears to splash down on her tender cheeks. But telling the truth is part and parcel of parenting, and children need parenting like a burger needs a bun.

Despite a minimum of 12 years of education, few of us receive the least bit of enlightenment as to how to parent a child. First offspring are usually born when we are still in our 20s, still grappling with questions of identity, still in the green stages of marital relationships. Functionally, young adults are still struggling with unresolved issues of late adolescence, and very likely skirmishing with their own issues of self-discipline, never mind disciplining a child.

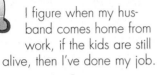

Wisdom of the Ages

I figure when my husband comes home from work, if the kids are still alive, then I've done my job.

—Roseanne Barr

Discipline. The word frightens many. It's often thought to be a punishment. But it's not. Discipline is structure. Children need it in order to learn and understand the order of things. Without offering them that gift of structure, which leads to self-control, they will be as lost as babes in the woods.

But when parenting takes the shape of a totalitarian regime, with equal treatment meted out for all, the opportunity of finding out, in very personal terms, who your children are is lost. Whatever values you wish to instill in your offspring, you must get to know them if you hope to be effective. As with any intimate relationship, this requires that you listen to them, respect them, admit when you're wrong, be firm when you know you're right, and show courage in your convictions. This will raise your family AQ.

If you don't encourage independence in your children—allowing them to pick their own clothes, for example, or cook their own breakfast—you're not going to have a very mature family AQ.

For the housewife with no interest outside her home and family, the growing independence of children can feel almost threatening. Anxious about her impending loss of identity, the mother might strive to keep the child dependent upon her in ways that can cripple the young one's chances of achieving self-reliance. Do you do your child's homework rather than helping him solve the problems himself? Have you settled disputes for your child rather than mediating a resolution between her and the others involved? These may seem like loving gestures, but in not allowing the child to work out such matters herself, it stunts her growth and development.

On the other side of the spectrum is too much independence—an "I don't need anyone" mentality. Some self-sufficiency is good, of course, but a strict diet of it handicaps a child: how can children learn to work with others, be a part of a team, if they're only taught to "do it yourself"?

Interdependence is the dynamic of being mutually responsible to and sharing a common set of principles with others. That is what encourages children to be cooperative, to listen to and respect others' approaches. Parents who encourage interdependence in their children are more likely to be included as part of the extended family when their children marry and have families of their own. A mature family AQ will surely arise from a family who is interdependent.

The most graceful and productive way for a mother to encourage inter-dependence in her offspring is to find some independence for herself. Whether it's teaching, typing, or tap dancing, a mother who has interests of her own is the best kind of model a child can have.

As the years roll by, mid-lifers will find themselves no longer the much-needed protectors of small children. In fact, parents of adolescents and young adults find that their progeny resents overprotectiveness. If a shift in the relationship doesn't occur, a rift will.

How Many Candles?

Despite a serious chronic disorder, this retired dentist stays physically fit with daily jogs, a good diet, and strict medical regime (medical AQ 28, physical fitness AQ 39), but he doesn't work at keeping his brain fit (brain AQ 49)—no challenging games, no writing, no continuing education, though he does read a fair amount and listen to music daily. His self-image is sturdy (self-image AQ 69) and his spiritual life is strong (spiritual AQ 70). Father of three and grandfather of nine, he is very close with his family (family AQ 62) and has a good relationship with his wife, with whom he shares regular activities, private time, and decision-making (significant other AQ 39). He stays very connected with his friends and his leisure time is well spent (social AQ 44). His true age is 59. His chronological age: 76. Considering his medical condition, this genarian has some amazing AQs and an enviable true age. But he could work on reaching out more to the community and being less reliant on family.

"So many people concentrate only on their children," an older mother said. "When they leave the nest, the mother jumps on the bottle, has a nervous breakdown, or goes wild." When this woman's two children, who she raised by herself, reached 21, she sat them down and said, "I've taught you everything I know. I don't know anything else. The three of us have been on my brain all these years. Now you've got to get off my brain. I would hope that what I've taught you has been good; it was the best I could do, and I hope you will take it and do something with it."

Siblings: Oh, Brother, Oh, Sister!

Siblings. They can be the best of friends, and they can be the worst of friends. No other peer can have as deep and thorough an understanding of your personal history as can your siblings. If you've emerged from a strong, bonded family, the friendship of your brothers and sisters can be among the most valued relationships of your lifetime.

Like parents, brothers and sisters have their major influence on each other during the first six years of life. When you're young, unless a lone child, you are either somebody's kid brother or sister, a person to be teased, prodded, and terrorized, and/or another's older sibling, who must be responsible and exemplary—and resents the younger like hell for the imposition. If you're in-betweeners in families with more than two children, you play both roles. The varying degrees of affection and hostility, of control and permissiveness, affects how you interrelate in later years. It makes a lasting imprint on your personality.

Optimize Your AQ

Childhood competitiveness and hostility, tempered with affection and goodwill, can actually strengthen character and the ability to relate well with others. Teasing can help thicken children's skin so they're better equipped to do battle with the world in later years. Sharing, so often resented, socializes children in ways that make them acceptable to the civilized world. Tender affection enables children to later open their hearts to relationships beyond those of blood relations.

In one family of three adult sisters, the middle one often cringed when observing how uptight the youngest sister would get whenever she asked her a series of questions—the subject matter was immaterial. The middle sister would ask herself, "Am I being authoritative? Is the tone of my voice patronizing?" It concerned her, for other than this particular dynamic, the two shared a wonderful relationship. She asked her husband and friends if they noticed a superiority in her manner when she interacted with her younger sister; they did not. But they didn't have the sisters' history. It could be something so subtle, so particular to their relationship, that only the younger would recognize it.

These early relationship patterns will follow you throughout your life. You need to be sensitive to them. As long as you're aware of them, as long as you refrain from being reactive to such a degree that they interfere with the basic foundation of the relationship, you can come out on top. Such a mature attitude will raise up the family AQ.

The Changing Family

With second and third marriages becoming commonplace, society has been more accepting of the concept of "blended families." They have become more acceptable. There may be children from each marriage. Many such blended families are finding new strengths and friendships in these extended circles, harkening back to yesteryear's larger families.

The family AQ is a difficult one to assess. There are so many subjective dynamics to take into account. The solidity of all your various relationships with the members of your immediate as well as extended family is the overriding factor. But looking at the component parts of those relationships is essential, too.

> **Wisdom of the Ages**
>
> Human beings are the only creatures who allow their children to come back home.
>
> —Bill Cosby

Are activities segregated by age group? If you live far away from the older parents, are there older friends who might serve as surrogates in family activities? Does affection abound among family members, or are demonstrations of love—kissing, hugging, verbal declarations—very limited or entirely off-limits?

Is there some activity enjoyed by the entire family? Family unity can be enhanced when family members participate in a shared activity, such as caring for the backyard garden or working toward and saving up for a family vacation.

Ask yourself the following questions when reviewing the level of maturity of your family AQ:

- Have the parents staked all their interests and energy in their offspring, or have they wisely anticipated the inevitable leave-taking of their young by establishing new interests and activities?

- As older parents, do you find yourself meddling in the affairs of your adult children? What can you offer in the way of a mature friendship with your grownup sons and daughters?

- Have you come to terms with old resentments with your brothers and sisters?

- As adult children, have you developed a more mature relationship with your parents, or do you still behave like Mama's little girl or Daddy's good boy? Have you forgiven your parents for childhood injuries? Have you learned to appreciate the true gifts your parents gave, expressing to them your gratitude and passing on those gifts to your own children?

As an adult, your may find yourself living far apart from your siblings and your parents—perhaps in another city or state. But if you've come from solid beginnings, geographical distance will not abate the affection and connection you feel.

The Least You Need to Know

- "Blended families" are the new extended families.
- Grownup siblings can be the best of friends.
- Parent-child relationships must change with the years.
- Young children need parameters and discipline from their parents.
- Affection flows freely in strong families.

Chapter **13**

Social True Age

In This Chapter

- ◆ Optimizing your social true age
- ◆ Developing friendships
- ◆ Keeping yourself well-rounded with hobbies
- ◆ Nurturing the child within

It's easy to underestimate the power of a touch, a smile, a kind word, a listening ear, an honest compliment, or the smallest act of caring, all of which have the potential to turn a life around. People come into your life for a reason, a season, or a lifetime. Embrace them all equally! Your social AQ is the outward you—how you relate to others, the quality of your friendships, and how you spend your leisure time.

Your Social True Age Quiz

1. What age group do you relate to most comfortably?

    B. Older than myself

    C. Younger than myself

    D. Around the same age as me

    E. Prefer a variety of ages

    F. It doesn't matter

2. What kind of people does your circle of friends consist of?

    C. Mixed ages, similar economic status

    F. Similar age group, but mixed economic status

    E. Mixed ages and economic status

    B. Similar in age and economic status

3. Do you have friends who you consider to be very close?

    A. None

    F. One to two

    H. Three to five

    D. Six to ten

    B. More than ten

4. How do you feel about your circle of friends?

    C. Somewhat unfulfilling

    B. Very unfulfilling

    H. Very fulfilling

    E. Somewhat fulfilling

5. How easily do you make new friends?

    D. Easily

    B. With great difficulty

    E. Fairly well, but not without effort

    A. Can't at all

    C. Not interested in doing so

6. How do you consider yourself to be?

    F. A friendly, outgoing person

    B. A loner; I keep to myself

    G. Receptive but reserved

    B. Painfully shy

    E. Unreceptive and/or cautious

7. In public places (stores, restaurants), do you make a personal connection with the personnel about anything outside of their job?

    F. Almost always

    B. Hardly ever

    E. Often, if I'm in a good mood

    D. Only if I have a complaint

8. How would you evaluate your leisure time?

    F. A bit too much of it, but well spent

    D. Not enough of it, but well spent

    E. Just the right amount, well spent

    B. A bit too much of it, and poorly spent

    A. Not enough of it, and poorly spent

    C. Just the right amount, but poorly spent

9. Which comes closest to your usual "night-out" activity?

    D. Going out to dinner alone or with spouse

    C. Watching TV with friends

    F. Going out to an event with friends

    A. Don't go out

    E. Gathering with friends for conversation, music, games, etc.

10. After dinner, how do you usually spend the bulk of your evening?

    D. Doing office work

    C. Watching television

    E. Doing domestic chores, home projects

    G. Reading, working on a hobby, computer surfing, etc.

    F. Talking on the phone with friends

    G. Usually out with friends, entertainment, etc.

11. How often do you think about your friends when you're not with them?

    C. Always

    F. Often

    D. Sometimes

    A. Rarely or never

12. How often do you attend social clubs, book groups, etc?

    H. Once a week

    E. Once a month

    F. Twice a month

    D. Five or six times a year

    J. Rarely or never

Scoring

Here's how to score your quiz:

1. Write in the letter for each answer in the "Letter" column.

2. Using the "Letter Values" list, find the value of points for each letter and write that number in the "Points" column.

3. Add up the points and write the total in the corresponding space.

4. Write in the *number of answers* you responded to for the section in the corresponding space and divide that number into the sum of points.

The result is your social true age!

Letter Values

A = 5 B = 15 C = 25 D = 35 E = 45 F = 55 G = 65 H = 75 I = 85 J = 95

Social True Age		
	Letter	Points
1.		
2.		
3.		
4.		
5.		
6.		
7.		
8.		
9.		
10.		
11.		
12.		
Total		
÷ #?s		
AQ		

Interpreting Your Score

Friends are lifelines to the world of sociability. Without them, life would feel cloistered. Friends offer a special kind of comfort and under-standing, as different from family support as it is essential. Friends invoke you to participate when you might not otherwise do so. They provide companionship, without which you couldn't play tennis or have parties. They perform tasks ranging from surrogate father or mother confessor, to watering the plants and feeding the cat when you're away on vacation. Friends help you get out of yourself. They are essential to a mature social AQ.

People with a mature social AQ are actively engaged in a social life with many interests and people. If your AQ is in the 40 to 50 range, your social life is probably at an optimum level. Under 30 or over 60, you might want to review the questions to see why your AQ is less than desirable.

The Importance of Friends

Making and maintaining friends is a lively and ongoing process. Old friends might move away, and while we might stay in touch, there is now a gaping hole in our daily social life until we develop new friend-ships. As we develop new interests, we might get hungry for new and different friends.

Children make friends quite readily. School is a perfect setup for mak-ing friends: there they are, learning together, struggling together, play-ing at recess together, and trying to buck a system together—peers, all. In addition, youngsters do not have the complex system of discrimina-tion that comes with maturity, so almost anyone will do as a friend.

How Many Candles?

A busy psychotherapist with almost as many grandchildren as she has fingers, this eldest daughter has a close relationship with all her family members (family AQ 46). Wonderfully fit (physical fitness AQ 24), she swims laps and does stretches daily, has a yellow belt in kick-boxing, and watches her diet. Her community AQ is solid (59) as she votes in all elections, does volunteer work weekly, and keeps up with political and cultural events. Her inner-life AQs are quite mature (self-image 83, spiritual 66, and future 86). She has a wide, satisfying circle of friends with whom she shares good times and entertainment (social AQ 46). Her true age is 57. Her chronological age: 70. This genarian has found a healthy, viable balance with a rich, full life.

But as you grow older and gain history, your friends become irreplace-able. You're willing to accept their faults because their attributes have become all the more dear to you. And because you've become more discriminating, it can be much harder to accept new people into your life. Except you must, if you're to enjoy friendships—and there's nary a soul who doesn't need them.

What are the ingredients of a solid friendship?

- ◆ Trustworthiness
- ◆ Being there to lend a hand—or an ear
- ◆ Sharing good times
- ◆ Being able to unburden yourself
- ◆ Common interests
- ◆ Shared basic values

Friendships require constant input and flexibility. Many adults complain that it is too hard to make new friends, so they just rely on chance. Of course, chance may bring rewarding friendships. But it is a rather passive attitude. Better to actively seek out friendships than leave it to chance. But how?

Clearly, you must expose yourself to groups of people where the potential for friendship exists. Becoming active in groups tailored to your interests is a great way to make that happen. Love nature? Join a birdwatchers group. Passionate about politics? Get involved with your political party, Common Cause, or the Women's League of Voters. Want to be fluent in French? Join a French club. Whatever your interests are, there are clubs and organizations populated with people who have common interests with you.

Wisdom of the Ages

Everyone wants to ride with you in the limo, but what you need is someone who will take the bus with you when the limo breaks down.

—Oprah Winfrey

The Art of Listening

If there was one thing and one thing only that you could do for a friend and you chose to listen, that would be the greatest gift you could possibly give. Not all the running of errands, babysitting, introductions, or even all the chicken soup in the world can take the place of a friend's receptive ear.

For some people, the art of listening comes naturally. For most, however, it is a skill that needs to be developed and honed.

Being an Active Listener

A good listener needs to know how to put herself in a receptive frame of mind—no judgment, no do-gooder responses, no solutions—just an open well, there to receive your friend's worries. The objective is to understand where your friend is coming from. As often as not, that's all a friend needs.

When your friend says she wants to talk, let her tell you everything she has to say before asking any questions. Interrupting the flow can short-circuit thought patterns. Encourage her to continue by using nonverbal or minimally verbal responses, like nodding or shaking your head, clucking your tongue in sympathy, murmuring "Uh-huh," "Really," "Go on," "What then?"

Once she's run out of steam, if you sense there is more to tell, ask some probing questions based on what you've just heard:

- ◆ "You said he stomped into the bedroom and slammed the door. What did he do then?"

- ◆ "How did you feel when she screamed, 'I hate you'?"

- ◆ "What did the doctor say after he gave you the diagnosis?"

These questions are inquisitive, not emotive or judgmental. You're not trying to stoke the fire here, just get your friend to talk so you can really know what's going on.

Mirroring

While you're listening, try to mirror your friend. If his energy is low and his speech reticent, respond at the same pace and in a similar tone. Conversely, if he's talking a mile a minute, don't respond so slowly that he throws up his hands with impatience. As an empathetic listener, you want to encourage your friend to keep talking.

Checkups

Once you think you've gotten all the information, check in to be certain you understand what your friend has been telling you. Communication can be difficult in the best of times, but it is more so when someone is upset. Instead of making assumptions, check out your understanding of the situation. Here are examples:

- ◆ "It sounds like you're having a really hard time telling your mother to stop telling you how to raise your kids. Is that right?"

- ◆ "So you're thinking she's really serious about leaving you, is that right?"

- ◆ "Are you telling me the doctor thinks there is no alternative to surgery?"

If you get confirmation, the conversation can progress from there. But if your friend says, "No, that's not what I meant at all," tell your friend you're sorry. You're trying to understand. "Tell me again, and give me a different example. I really want to hear what you're going through." Soon enough, you'll find you're both on the same page.

Even if the problem seems slight to you, do not make light of your friend's worries, else you will lose your status as a confidante.

While you may dream of rescuing your friends from their various pains and dilemmas, in the final analysis, the most empowering thing you can do is to encourage them to solve their own problems. Your goal as a friend is not to make them do what you say, but to help them figure out their own solutions.

Ask pertinent questions, like, "All right now, what could you do about this matter?" Suggest that it may help to break down the problem into smaller ones and work to solve them. Encourage realistic, achievable goals. Follow up with a phone call. See how your friend is doing.

Reevaluating Friendships

As you grow older and you attain more stability in your life, your interests turn outward more and more. Companions may take on added importance, particularly as children leave the nest or you find yourself living alone. Where once you planned vacations around your immediate family, now you may join three or four friends for a week's outing. Where Saturdays may once have consisted of a day at the zoo or an amusement park, now a few friends might attend a concert together or play bridge. The more experiences you share, the more you come to know one another, and the more real you can be with your friends, enabling you to drop the various facades demanded by daily exigencies. It's relaxing; it's revivifying. You can get to the nitty-gritty with a friend as you can with no other person.

A friendship that lies fallow, however, will pull on you, weigh you down, and hold back your personal growth. Friendships need to be lively things, full of the stuff of life. They may be brand new or decades old, but if they aren't spry then they are lifeless. A friendship that affords no stimulation of the mind, of the spirit, or at least of the body—like a good tennis partner or jogging mate—is of little use and would best be put behind you. Instead, put your energy into newer relationships, bringing them into the foreground.

Wisdom of the Ages

A grandmother was telling her little granddaughter what her own childhood was like: "We used to skate outside on a pond. I had a swing made from a tire; it hung from a tree in our front yard. We rode our pony. We picked wild raspberries in the woods." The little girl was wide-eyed, taking this in. At last she said, "I sure wish I'd gotten to know you sooner!"

Everyone changes and grows, but rarely at the same rate or in similar directions. Despite the fact that you may have outgrown a friendship, you might be uncomfortable letting go of it. You don't want to hurt anyone, but you can feel trapped. You need to find a way of letting go, allowing the friendship to drift apart gently. Try some simple, unemotive actions, like being unable to take a call, having to cancel an engagement, not showing eagerness at setting up new ones. You have to take care of yourself; you want to use your time and energy for engaging with someone who is more stimulating and fulfilling.

This is not meant to suggest that old friends be discarded like old shoes. To the contrary: old friends are often the best. But the texture of some of your relationships is going to change as your priorities in life alter. It is up to you to continually evaluate how well the potential of each friendship is being fulfilled.

If a friend has hurt you in some way, instead of pretending like it didn't happen, which will eventually ruin the friendship, talk to your friend about it. Perhaps she wasn't aware of the slight, or how deeply it cut. Even if she was aware of it, the process of forgiveness cannot begin without both of you acknowledging the situation. James Baldwin once wrote, "You cannot fix what you will not face." Face each other. Acknowledge that harm has been done. Work at forgiveness (it doesn't happen overnight). If the friendship has value, it is worth working to preserve it. Those with mature social AQs know that.

Spontaneity is a valuable ingredient in any relationship. Spur of the moment goings-on can often lead to memorable experiences. But those activities we anticipate, carefully plan, and look forward to, are as fundamental to a full and rewarding relationship as are those of a moment's fancy. Creating rituals that include friends is a great asset in maintaining friendships.

From the New Year's Gala to class reunions to the annual Fourth of July picnic, friends need to find times and structures within which they can be together. This is especially so for those whose preoccupation with career and house-holding can limit social life.

Leisure Time Activities

What kind of entertainment do you prefer? What adventures do you anticipate? What you do with vacations, evenings, and weekends? Americans spend an average of four to six hours a day watching television, and three to four hours daily on the Internet at home. Most folks have a good deal of excess time on their hands. Weekends may find you lolling around for hours with the Sunday paper and more television.

How do you spend your leisure time? Check all that apply:

- ❏ Visiting the homes of neighbors, friends, and relatives
- ❏ Dining out
- ❏ Going to the movies
- ❏ Walks or hikes at parks
- ❏ Attending sports events
- ❏ Attending live theater, and dance or musical concerts
- ❏ Going to museums
- ❏ Going to events at community or recreational centers
- ❏ Traveling to other countries
- ❏ Playing a sport

The more boxes you checked, the more mature your social AQ. Unless, that is, you're so overscheduled with engagements and activities that you're stressed out. Downtime is important, too; that "lolling around" mentioned earlier can sometimes be a great de-stressor.

Participatory sports—jogging, bicycling, skiing, or tennis—are excellent ways to spend leisure time. They stimulate not only the body, but also the spirit, because the confidence achieved by growing expertise and accomplishment can make the spirit soar. And they strengthen bonds with your buddies.

Hobbies are usually a more solitary pursuit, but they are equally important to your health as a social being—it's important to enjoy your own company. Hobbies bring relief from the day's obligations. They also provide mental stimulation. And there's not a one of them that doesn't have a club or association where you can share the snags and triumphs with similarly interested folks.

Some hobbies are meant for just one pair of hands, but several can be group-oriented, such as nature walks or quilting. While solitary creative work is important and rewarding, it's as important to be engaged in sociable activities.

How Many Candles?

An executive assistant with a furniture chain, this twice-divorced mother of two toddlers was raised in a medium-sized town and now lives in her own home in a small city. Having a romantic bent, her singleness frustrates her (singleness AQ 33). Fortunately she is very close with her parents and sisters, though she confesses that she spends perhaps a little too much time with them (family AQ 52). She is very happy in her work, where she enjoys an ample income and sees room for advancement (financial AQ 56). While she has an interest in politics and cultural happenings, she isn't at all involved in community groups or does she do volunteer work (community AQ 42). But she has a very satisfying circle of friends around her own age with whom she loves to get together for good times. However, she doesn't belong to any social clubs and spends most evenings watching TV (social AQ 49). Her true age is 48. Her chronological age: 33.

Clearly a mature young woman, she could do herself a favor by getting more involved in her community and relying a little less on her family. Such action would very likely raise her singleness AQ and lower her social AQ, although the latter is certainly optimal now.

Personality Review

In Chapter 7, you explored your self-image AQ, a singular excursion illustrating how you see yourself. Now it's time to discover how others see you.

Do you take the time to look deeply into the mirror of your friends' reflections of you? Are you patient and tolerant with those who are slower to grasp concepts than you might be? Are you hostile and defensive with those who are quicker and more demanding? Do you impose your priorities on others, feeling impelled to put down any but your own values and choices? Or do you delight in the variety, the differences that abound among people?

Look to Others for a View of Yourself

Those of you who have taken drama classes may remember three principal rules for creating a character:

◆ Look for what the character has to say about himself.

- Look for what the playwright has to say about the character.

- Look for what the other characters have to say about a particular character.

To some extent, you are your own playwright, composing the story of your life. And these same rules for creating a character apply. And it's that third rule that can hang you up. It's all too easy to block out the little reminders that are put to you daily in a steady stream of reactions and responses from others. Rather than look to yourself, you claim, like the sodden barfly, "I'm not drunk—it's the rest of the world that's spinning."

Let Your Hair Down

Another avenue toward social development is to shed the skin of "adult behavior" when you're among friends, and recognize that you need to express the many ages within you. The child within needs to get out and play: display it, enjoy it, and share it with those close to you, just as you do your adult self. Even adults need role models, so being around younger people can help you keep in touch with your own inner child.

Whether or not you consider yourself to be master of your fate, you are in charge of what you do with it and how you feel about it. Scrooge, of Dickens's *A Christmas Carol*, no doubt had a very immature social AQ. He didn't share his largess with others, and he never cracked a smile. Smiling, laughing—the gift of doing so at one's own expense and allowing others to do so as well—is literally a gift of life.

The late political journalist and professor Norman Cousins once wrote, "Laughter is a form of internal jogging. It moves your internal organs around. It enhances respiration. It is an igniter of great expectations." It has been proven that laughter stimulates the glands to produce ACTA, which is a healing chemical, a healing hormone. It can actually help sick people become well, which is what Cousins was writing about. If laughter helps get you back to normal when you're under the weather, think what it can do when you're up to par! Make sure you have friends with whom you laugh a lot.

Be Adventurous

How many people live like overfed apartment-imprisoned cats, never venturing out, never nosing around, never taking risks? They're safe—and stagnant. They've allowed themselves to be cowed by media portrayals of unsafe neighborhoods, by corporate threats of financial insecurity (save it now so you'll be taken care of later), by government oppressiveness that makes it impossible to do, oh, so many things: hike off the beaten path, raise chickens in the city, work until you're 100. So what can you do about it?

This is not meant to suggest you break city ordinances and start raising chickens on your apartment balcony! But you could learn a new skill, something you've always wanted to do, something that feels daring to you—like belly dancing or kick-boxing. You could go someplace you've always wanted to go to; it doesn't have to be far. There are New Yorkers who have never been to Ellis Island, South Dakotans who have never visited Mt. Rushmore, Floridians who have never boated through the Everglades. Tourists often get to see more of a city than its denizens.

Setting off the mainspring of adventure catapults you into more meaningful, intimate friendships. Your leisure time will become more purposeful. Your personality, like a peacock's tail feathers, will fan out in unsuspected colors that dazzle and energize. You will be on the road to achieving a mature social AQ, one that gives you the opportunity to reshape yourself, your direction, your friendships, your goals, and your fantasies.

The Least You Need to Know

- Good friendships are essential to a healthy life.
- The best thing you can do for a friend is to listen.
- Pay attention to what friends have to tell you about yourself.
- Developing hobbies is a great way to meet like-minded people and fulfill your own creativity.
- Life should be an adventure—it's up to you to make it one.

Chapter 14

Financial True Age

In This Chapter

- ◆ Optimizing your financial true age
- ◆ Putting joy into your work
- ◆ Opening up your options
- ◆ Preparing for new work
- ◆ Evaluating your income

In America, we have what many call the Protestant or Puritan work ethic—work hard, sacrifice, never give up, and you'll be rewarded. This attitude toward work was unknown until the sixth century when St. Benedict posted the following rule at his monastery at Monte Cassino: "Idleness is the enemy of the soul. And therefore, at fixed times, the brothers ought to be occupied in manual labor, and, again at fixed times, in sacred reading." The dictum was clear that one had to work if one were to be "saved," whether it was necessary for one's survival or not. And so began society's compulsion to work, work, work.

Your Financial True Age Quiz

1. How do you feel in your present line of work?

   F. Extremely satisfied

   E. Very satisfied

   D. Moderately satisfied

   C. Slightly unsatisfied

   B. Very dissatisfied

   A. Extremely dissatisfied

2. In your work, how do you see yourself?

   F. Gaining advancement

   E. Keeping the status quo

   C. Losing status

   D. Changing line of work

3. What have you done to advance your profession in your post-school years?

   A. Haven't done anything

   E. Attended a few classes or seminars

   G. Went back for a degree

   F. Learned a new skill

   D. Kept abreast by studying professional journals

4. Does your household income cover your expenses?

   G. Yes, amply

   E. Yes, adequately

   C. Yes, minimally

   A. No, and I don't know what to do about it

   B. No, I must rely on family assistance, alimony, credit, etc.

5. Which of the following statements best describes your economic circumstance?

    E. Just manage to pay my bills

    C. Live on credit somewhat

    F. Always save a little something

    B. Deeply in debt

    G. Invest in mutual funds, stocks, property

6. What are your plans with regard to retirement?

    G. Don't plan to retire at this time

    F. Will retire at expected age (62–70)

    D. Will retire as soon as possible

    C. Don't want to retire; am being forced to

    E. Don't know when to retire

7. What are your plans after retirement?

    G. Attend school or start up a new career or business

    C. Don't know

    D. Just relax and socialize

    H. Don't plan to retire

    I. Devote myself to community

    F. Pursue hobbies and recreational service activities

8. Aside from Social Security, how have you provided for your retirement income?

    H. Interest from savings and investments

    G. A strong pension plan

    B. Will rely on another's income

    A. No provisions made

9. If your present line of work is homemaker, which of the following would most apply when your child/ren grow older or leave home?

F. Go to school or take a job

G. Do volunteer work

C. Relax and take it easy

B. Don't know what I'll do

D. Continue keeping the home for my spouse

10. If you were to lose your mate for any reason, what would you most likely do?

E. Hire help to manage house or accounts

F. Manage household duties myself

B. Find another mate as soon as possible

D. Go to live with a family member

G. Find friend(s) to live with

C. Don't know what I'd do

Scoring

Here's how to score your quiz:

1. Write in the letter for each answer in the "Letter" column.

2. Using the "Letter Values" list, find the value of points for each letter and write that number in the "Points" column.

3. Add up the points and write the total in the corresponding space.

4. Write in the *number of answers* you responded to for the section in the corresponding space and divide that number into the sum of points.

The result is your financial true age!

Letter Values

A = 5 B = 15 C = 25 D = 35 E = 45 F = 55 G = 65 H = 75 I = 85 J = 95

Financial True Age		
	Letter	Points
1.		
2.		
3.		
4.		
5.		
6.		
7.		
8.		
9.		
10.		
Total		
÷ #?s		
AQ		

Interpreting Your Score

Whether you're installing the motherboard into a computer, creating pie charts for a stock-holder's meeting, or serving food in a restaurant, your job encompasses just one part of a much bigger process. It's important to feel you're an integral part of that process, to feel connected to your work. Without some feeling of connection, your work week will sap you of energy. As important, of course, is earning enough money to at least meet your financial obligations, preferably with some left over for savings and for fun!

Those of you who enjoy your work and who are not worried about finances will find you have a financial AQ at least over 40. If it's under that, especially if it's under 30, it behooves you to review the questions and see what you can do to change your work and financial life. That could mean a new job or career or budgeting yourself in a way that's more in keeping with your means.

Job Satisfaction

Work must have life to it if you are to remain interested and engaged. When you consider that most people spend about 40 percent of their adult lives at work, it's easy to see why it's so important to have some joy during that time. Sometimes the constant striving for "more" so many are driven to—more success, more status, more money—whether on the corporate ladder or the assembly line, may not bring contentment and fulfillment. In fact, because you may feel you're losing contact with other parts of your life—relationships with family and friends, everyday activities—you may actually feel a sense of discontent. Getting more out of life is more important than getting more money, status, or power. What you truly need on the job is satisfaction.

Make Work Fun

Work can be made into play, or at least a pleasurable procedure. By learning to be malleable, adjusting your goals and expectations, you can find satisfaction on the job. By discovering ways to put zest back into your labor, you can experience satisfaction and vigor in your work. How do you do that?

For years, teams of garbage collectors would race down the narrow cobbled streets of New Orleans's French Quarter. As they removed overflowing trash cans from below street-level repositories, emptied them into an enormous bin truck that followed at their heels, and then replaced the cans in the deep sidewalk wells, the collectors moved so fast they appeared to be flying. When a group of visitors on a tour of the city asked their guide why the garbage collectors were racing, the guide told them, "They've always done it like that, as far as I can remember. It's a game with them: teams race against other teams to see who gets back to the plant first."

These men had put zest back into what most would regard as a dreary routine. Their job did not wither them; instead, it invigorated them.

Most of you can no longer literally run in your work, but you can challenge yourself by developing speed with your skills, your efficiency, your mind.

If speed is out of the question in your line of work, there are other ways to add some spice to your daily routine. The inimitable Gertrude Stein once said, "Counting is the religion of this generation; it is its hope and its salvation." Almost everyone loves to count. Counting is a way of measuring your competence, of feeling you've accomplished something. This tendency to tabulate can be used to your advantage at work: counting time, counting pieces, or counting lists of things to do can instill you with a sense of competition that injects your labor with liveliness. At a script service in Hollywood, typists gather in the break room at the end of the shift, sharing coffee and donuts to see who typed the most pages.

Or perhaps your work could enable you to let your mind drift. If you execute simple, repetitive tasks, let the monotony create a rhythmic background for a mind trip. At a manufacturing plant outside Los Angeles, one fellow in the plant sings, picking up the rhythm of the machines. At a Waffle House in Tallahassee, a waitress serenades the customers with her delightful voice.

Whether it be speed, competition, fantasy, introspection, philosophy, or song, finding joy in your work can replenish your soul.

Personalize Your Space

Make your work space as homey and comfortable as company policy will allow. Pictures of family, friends, and pets; a potted plant; a fun coffee mug; maxims and mantras; a comfortable chair: such personal touches bring warmth to your work. If you work for a large corporation, find out what social activities it sponsors and get involved: join the ball team; start up a book group that meets at lunch once a month; bug upper management to open a daycare center.

Let's say you've done everything a person could do to make your job more satisfying, and it still isn't working for you. You're at a point where you're convinced the only thing that's going to put joy in your work is to find another job, another career. Where do you begin?

Optimize Your AQ

Remember, you spend 40 percent of your time at work. Invest your creativity and energy into making it your home away from home.

Considering a Career Change

Be systematic when you're considering a career change. Before you start actively searching, take the following steps:

1. **Assess yourself.** Make a list of your skills, your aptitudes, your propensities. If you have a knack for mechanics and all things technical but you are not a terrific communicator, think about heading in the direction of computer technology, not hospitality services. Study your list.

2. **Make a plan.** Rather than going at a career change helter-skelter, write a mission plan for yourself. Know what you're looking for. Plan how to go about achieving your goals.

3. **Study the market.** Be sure you gear your search toward a market that is viable and not on the wane. The fields of education and health services, for example, are expanding. You can study trends at www.khake.com, a vocational information center.

4. **Write a resumé tailored to your audience.** Competition can be fierce in the marketplace. A professional presentation, focused and lucid, can make all the difference.

If you're having trouble figuring out the best direction for you, you might want to take the Myers/Briggs personality test (www.myersbriggs.org). Knowing your personality type can help you choose your first career, advance in your organization, or change careers. Myers/Briggs is a practical tool for investigating what works for you, then looking for and recognizing work that satisfies your preferences. A person with a preference for introversion, for example, may find he or she is happier doing research, while a person who prefers extraversion may favor a field with more interaction with people. The more you know about yourself, the more successful you can be at making the best choices for you.

Look at Your Options

There's a world of possibilities, for both men and women. "There are very few jobs that require a penis or a vagina," said the irrepressible civil rights lawyer Flo Kennedy. "All other jobs should be open to everybody." Women, in addition to the traditional jobs of teaching, nursing, and clerical work, are now plumbers, CEOs, and astronauts. Male teachers are needed in elementary schools; nursing is attracting many men these days. There are dozens of career-change clinics established to help you ascertain whether or not you should move on or stay put. Filled with ideas to stimulate your imagination, they lead you to mull over all kinds of possibilities.

Write a Resumé

Now about that resumé. Just as styles in fashion change over the years, so do styles in resumés. Yours must look up-to-the-minute and professional. You can hire a professional to do it, or you can do it yourself. There's plenty of help for that task, from books to free tips online at websites like www.how-to-write-a-resume.org and the similarly titled www.howtowritearesume.net. Just remember, if your resumé doesn't grab the hiring agent in the first 20 to 30 seconds, it goes into the trash bin.

Same goes for your cover letter. A cover letter is not a resumé. It has one purpose: to demonstrate that you meet or exceed the requirements listed in the job description. Keep it simple and factual. Let the company know that you're interested in the position, and are available to accept it. Don't get into salary requirements, family background, and that you love dogs. Information beyond the essential not only dilutes the core purpose of the cover letter, but it can be harmful to your chances.

Get Your Name Out There

Okay, now you're ready to pursue that career change. Start networking. It really is true that it often comes down to "who you know" when it comes to getting your perfect position. Most people get their jobs by networking. Of course, check out the classifieds. Be aware there are many career clinics that can steer you in the right direction. There are even services that will distribute your resumé for you to hundreds of potential employers: www.resumeblaster.com, www.forwardyourresume.com, www.resumeXposure.com, and www.resumedeliver.com. Be aware, however, that the spam approach disallows you from personalizing that cover letter. On the other hand, you can customize your profile and even target geographic areas. According to one article, more and more recruiters and employment agencies are turning to resumé distribution services to find suitable candidates for jobs in hundreds of industries.

Hone Your Skills

The more you educate yourself, the more you'll know about your work, and the more you will be able to offer to your employer and yourself. Skill is the whetstone upon which you may sharpen your vigor and imagination; it's the helium that can lift your spirits.

Don't be a Fred or Wilma Flintstone: get out there and learn the new technology. There are very few jobs these days that don't require computer knowledge, including software ranging from word processing to spreadsheets to databases to graphics.

You might need to get some training or go back to school. Where do you begin to know where to go? There is so much help waiting for you on the Internet. For example, www.careerexplorer.net has a terrific list of colleges, universities, and career-training schools. If you plug in the field that interests you and your zip code, it will lead you to campuses in your area as well as online programs in your field.

The costs of these courses varies widely, depending upon the facility, the length of time of the course, and the degree offered. At a public university, you should expect to pay anywhere between $110 and $300 per credit (most classes are 3 credits). What if you simply can't afford the costs of tuition? There are several options open to you in the way of student loans and grants. But the best place to start is with The Free Application for Federal Student Aid, or FAFSA (www.fafsa.ed.gov).

Wisdom of the Ages

> A handout distributed by Virginia Boyack, Ph.D., during a seminar at USC's School of Gerontology included this poem, titled "The Rocking Chair," written by an anonymous author:
>
> The rocking chair will be empty today.
> For Grandma is no longer in it.
> She's off in her car to her office or shop.
> And buzzes around every minute.
> No one can shove Grandma back on the shelf,
> She's versatile, thoughtful, dynamic.
> That isn't a pie in the oven, you know,
> Her baking today is ceramic.
> You won't see her trundling off early to bed.
> From her place in the warm chimney nook.
> Her typewriter clackity-clacks through the night,
> For Grandmother's writing a book.
> She isn't content with crumbs of old thought,
> With meager secondhand knowledge.
> So don't bring your mending for Grandma to do,
> For Grandma has gone back to college.

Self-Employment

Perhaps you've always dreamed of starting your own business. It isn't right for everybody. Look back at your self-assessment, and ask yourself these questions:

- Am I self-motivated?

- Am I disciplined?

- Am I a risk-taker, or does insecurity make me very anxious?

- Can I live with the financial ups and downs, or do I need to know exactly what's coming in each week?

- Can I afford to take the time to establish a new business?

- Do I have staying power?

If you can answer yes to those questions, self-employment may be the most satisfying path to follow. A little lateral thinking can come into play here. If you look to your life experiences, you may be able to harvest many possibilities for second and third careers—as consultants, nursery men, furniture-makers, and so on. Life is an education. And yours has prepared you for work, whether you know it or not. Look at these people who used their life experience to start new careers:

♦ The mother of a son afflicted with Down's Syndrome became deeply involved in her son's education, teaching him to walk, talk, and take care of himself, despite having been told he could never do those things. She became very involved in a pilot program for the handicapped as well as the PTA and other community organizations. She became a well-known figure in her town, and gained a great deal of experience working with public agencies. Years later, she opened her own daycare center.

♦ A woman married young and moved with her husband to Cuba, where she lived through Castro's takeover. Not long after, she returned to the States with her two children, divorced and penniless. An amateur historian of her homeland, she became very involved with the community, opening a tourist center.

♦ A 45-year-old Air Force retiree turned his hobby of collecting Indian artifacts into a viable business. He also learned foundry work while in the Air Force. Within a few years, he was doing castings for the Smithsonian Institution. After a few years, he sold his Indian artifacts and bought into a large gallery in Santa Fe.

♦ A woman who loved the arts worked as a customer service rep, selling season tickets and doing fundraising for theaters. Her boss encouraged her to run a season ticket drive herself. She started with a small client, and within two years she was her previous boss's biggest competitor—and friend.

There are lots of books that will help you kick-start your own business: *The Complete Idiot's Guide to Starting Your Own Business* is a great place to begin.

Keep an Open Mind

It is no longer unusual to see mayors who are 22, college presidents who are 30, retirees at 50, 70-year-old students, and even 85-year-old mothers who are caring for their 65-year-old children. Age is no longer a meaningful marker.

More and more people are taking a "serial career" approach to their work-life, in which they pursue a number of different careers within their lifetime. With longer life expectancies, the serial career can be a practical and attractive alternative.

These days more and more corporations are developing worker and family-friendly policies. If that is important to you, look for the following at any companies you are considering working for:

- Midlife sabbaticals, either job-related or not.

- Transferable pension plans, enabling you to move from one company to another without the risk of losing future security.

- Flexible work weeks: four 10-hour days, six 6-hour days, eight 48-hour weeks with every fifth week off, etc.

- Project-oriented hours: whenever you finish the job, the rest of the day could be yours.

- Telecommuting, which enables you to do some work at home.

- Child-care programs, either on site or off. Some companies even have breastfeeding rooms for nursing mothers.

- Maternity/Paternity Leave Policy, allowing mothers—and fathers—at least six weeks to be home with their newborns or a sick child.

- Wellness programs that provide on-site gyms where you can work out before lunch or on breaks. Some companies even offer classes from yoga to managing stress.

- Work/life programs that provide pet care, dry cleaning, psychologists, referral services—all the things so impossible to do when you have long work days.

- Educational programs that offer the skills you need for promotion and advancement.

Research the companies you'd like to work for to see how well they fit in with your goals and desires.

Midlife can be a prime time for a turnabout in work, when discontent with or the threat of losing a job looms. Consider the possibilities, not with a gloom-and-doom attitude, but with a sense of adventure and challenge. Look through the classified ads, call employment agencies or career counselors, take some classes, attend some seminars or conventions. Shake yourself up a little. It will stir up your mind in a way that prevents stagnation and presents new possibilities.

Look at your alternatives and consider the possibilities. If you're content where you are now, terrific. Stick with it. But what happens if, happy though you may be, you are forced into early retirement by company policy?

Money, Money, Money

Although money isn't everything, having enough money to pay your bills and set aside a retirement nest egg is essential for happiness. Success is so tied into making money that it's very difficult to separate one from the other.

Finances affect health, which affects the way you age. A study was made by life insurance analysts of 6,329 prominent professional and businessman who were listed in *Who's Who in America*. It revealed that, on the average, prominent men live longer than other men with similar occupations who were not prominent. It seems the old adage "success kills" is inaccurate.

Matthew Herper, in his article "Why the Rich Live Longer" (*Forbes* magazine, September 13, 2001) claims that "wealth and success … stave off death. In fact, the strain of not getting them may be what kills us." He continues to say that a lot of prior research has shown that "those who are higher on the social and economic food chain are also blessed with longer lives. Moreover, many researchers are beginning to reject theories that explain away the difference by noting that those with more money can afford better lives, including better housing, food and health care. Instead, many are turning to a psychological explanation: stress." The evidence began accumulating 20 years ago with a British medical survey of civil servants called the Whitehall Study. Robert Sapolsky, a neurobiologist at Stanford University, is a proponent of the idea that our social and economic position directly affects our susceptibility to any number of diseases, and ultimately the length of our lives.

How can you raise your economic status? Because there is a definite correlation between economics and life span, it would be wise to do everything you can to achieve that.

Of course, money is but one of many factors involved in life span. One 57-year-old man whose financial AQ was 52 was unemployed, although his annual income was still about $30,000. He had no dependent children and was happily married. Due to investments and savings and owning his own home, this man managed to come up with a strong financial AQ despite the fact that he earned a modest income.

It's interesting to note that while an adequate income does affect the financial AQ, a large income doesn't automatically give you a mature one. One 57-year-old editor/writer with an annual household income of more than $90,000 had a financial AQ of only 49—not that there's anything wrong with that, but considering how happy he was in his work and the comfortable income, it seemed off. Analyzing the quiz answers, the reasons weren't immediately apparent, but his response that he would have to rely on another's income in his retirement years prompted us to examine his demographic profile (demographics were requested of all solicited respondents). He was married for the second time. His earnings were exactly half of that $90,000, his current wife providing the other half. He had six children by his first wife, and while the youngest was now 19, no doubt the cost of their upbringing and schooling continued to drain much of his income.

When trying to up your economic status, the direct approach is often the swiftest: request a raise, ask for a bonus and/or promotion, or change jobs or careers. There is always the possibility of moonlighting, too. If you're spending most evenings watching TV and complaining about your bills as well as the programming, you might be better off working two or three nights a week, or taking classes that would ultimately upgrade your earning potential.

You can also reduce your expenses. Because the key factor in the influence of money on aging and health is having enough money to avoid stress, rather than having a lot of money, reducing expenses is yet another arrow in your quiver to aim for a mature financial AQ. Economizing is not only a sure way to raise your financial AQ, but, in terms of self-satisfaction, it is rewarding in and of itself.

Whatever your economic goals may be, don't put yourself out of the ballgame before you've even started. Set small, attainable goals. This is far healthier than setting such a big goal that you may have a heart attack before you achieve it.

Retirement and Financial Planning

Take a realistic look at your financial future: your Social Security will not, in all likelihood, be enough to support you. Do you have a pension plan where you work, or will your savings be adequate to handle your future needs? Can you continue working well into old age? What will you do when you retire? Are there alternative work programs for which you can begin to prepare now? Are you maintaining a lifestyle you can afford without duress? Do you have savings? These are important questions to ask yourself; their answers will partially regulate your financial AQ.

You've now asked yourself whether or not you like your work, whether you'd consider doing other work, what you would be willing to do to obtain it, and whether you've given any serious thought to your retirement years. These are essential questions in ascertaining your financial AQ. If, after completing the quiz, you found your financial AQ to be quite young, you should examine your present and future work life and financial status.

The Least You Need to Know

- Finding joy in your work is of the utmost importance.
- Look outside traditional employment practices to find what's right for you.
- Educating yourself by learning new skills increases your chances for advancement.
- Financial planning is essential to your well-being.

Chapter **15**

Community True Age

In This Chapter

- ◆ Optimizing your community true age
- ◆ Embracing your civic duties
- ◆ Improving your neighborhood
- ◆ Working with political-action committees
- ◆ Expanding your cultural horizons

Are you involved in community activities? Do you follow local, state, and national politics? What are your concerns with fashion and trends in the world of art, music, and lifestyles? Do you keep up with the times, or are you living in the past?

Your Community True Age Quiz

1. In what way are you active in civic causes?

    C. Vote, but nothing more

    E. Vote and contribute to causes

    B. Take no interest in civic causes

    G. Can't afford to contribute, but I vote and volunteer

    H. Vote, make contributions, do volunteer work

2. How often do you do volunteer work?

    H. Daily

    G. Weekly

    F. One to two times a month

    D. Only occasionally

    B. Never or hardly ever

3. In what way do you keep current with cultural and/or world events?

    F. Via daily mainstream and alternative media

    D. Weekly news magazines

    B. Don't keep at all current

    A. From friends and family

    E. Alternative news sources only

    G. A variety of sources on a daily basis

4. What is your interest in music, art, fashion, entertainment, etc.?

    C. Not at all interested

    E. Mildly interested

    B. It's my main focus

    G. Very interested

5. What is your interest in political issues and news of the day?

    C. Not at all interested

    E. Mildly interested

    B. It's my main focus

    G. Very interested

6. How often do you tend to analyze or try to figure out the motives or states of mind of community leaders and decision-makers?

   G. Often

   E. Sometimes

   C. Rarely or never

7. How often do you meet with community groups?

   H. Once a week

   G. Twice a month

   F. Once a month

   E. Five or six times a year

   B. Rarely or never

8. What is your involvement with activist or charitable organizations?

   G. Moderately active

   E. Occasionally get involved

   I. Deeply committed

   C. Not at all involved

9. What are your voting habits?

   E. Vote only in national elections

   C. Vote sporadically, when I remember

   I. Vote in all elections—local, state, national

   A. Don't vote or rarely vote

   G. Vote only in state and/or national elections

10. How often do you participate in community events?

    G. At least once every month or two

    I. More than once a month

    E. Once or twice a year

    A. I never participate

Scoring

Here's how to score your quiz:

1. Write in the letter for each answer in the "Letter" column.

2. Using the "Letter Values" list, find the value of points for each letter and write that number in the "Points" column.

3. Add up the points and write the total in the corresponding space.

4. Write in the *number of answers* you responded to for the section in the corresponding space (the one that looks like this: ÷ #?s) and divide that number into the sum of points.

The result is your community true age!

Letter Values

A = 5 B = 15 C = 25 D = 35 E = 45 F = 55 G = 65 H = 75 I = 85 J = 95

Community True Age		
	Letter	**Points**
1.		
2.		
3.		
4.		
5.		
6.		
7.		
8.		
9.		
10.		
Total		
÷ #?s		
AQ		

Interpreting Your Score

A fully lived life broadens its circle beyond family and friends to the wider community. Life is filled with varied and numerous contacts with hundreds of shopkeepers, coworkers, repairpersons, doctors, accountants, delivery folks, and neighbors. Just like you, those individuals are affected by the political and civic goings-on of the nation and the local community. To achieve a mature community AQ, it is necessary to be engaged with the members and organizations of your community.

Those of you who belong to local chapters of social service and political organizations and who actively work to achieve their goals are far more likely to have a mature community AQ, somewhere in the 50s or 60s, than those who do not. Those of you who attend exhibits at the museum; go to concerts; and read up on current trends in fashion, architecture, and such will also boost your AQ up to the 40s or 50s. But it is those who do all the above, and who are active citizens in local, state, and national elections, who will achieve the most mature community AQs, often in their 70s or even their 80s.

Civic Duties

Many Americans consider civic involvement to be an optional leisure activity. Anyone who thinks that will certainly not achieve a very mature community AQ. As citizens, you have an obligation, beyond your own fireside, to give aide and support to your fellow humans. That is what elevates us as a society. But beyond this moral compulsion to help others, there are many other good reasons why it is important to be an engaged member of your community and to volunteer your services:

- ◆ It feels good.
- ◆ It strengthens family ties, especially when done as a family unit.
- ◆ It cultivates a sense of responsibility (especially important for children).
- ◆ It brings you in touch with people of different backgrounds, ethnicities, and economic groups.

♦ It can help you develop leadership and other skills.

♦ It can be a conduit to new career opportunities.

♦ It reinforces your commitment to your community.

Why should you worry about your community? Isn't it enough to take care of your own home, your own family, your own backyard?

You can't help but be concerned about your community, because you are connected to it in dozens of ways: the infrastructure that enables you to get water from your tap, turn on the lights, make a phone call, drive to the supermarket, take the bus to work, send the kids to school, borrow books from the library, call the police or the fire department when there's an emergency—all these and more would not be possible without a strong community. If the community falls apart, your life will suffer. Communities—and nations—work better when their citizens participate.

Volunteer Your Time

Volunteering doesn't have to take a lot of time. Look at your own schedule and availability. You can volunteer once or twice a year, once or twice a month, or every day. Once you make a commitment, people are going to be counting on you, so before you offer your services, you need to know your time availability.

There are three basic ways you can become an active member of your community:

♦ Donate time

♦ Share your skills and talents

♦ Give money

Volunteering is rewarding if it is geared toward your interests. If you offer your services to an organization that doesn't galvanize your own interests, you will tire of it all too soon.

If you have enough money to sponsor a little league team or buy land for a neighborhood playground or green area, great. But the real gift of giving is your time and your talent. The beauty of it is, you can match your interests with the needs of your community and find the perfect marriage. Here are just a few of the myriad possibilities:

◆ Help build a local home with Habitat for Humanity.

◆ Read and record books for the blind.

◆ Cook, serve food, or clean up at a local food bank or soup kitchen.

◆ Join a mentoring program at your neighborhood school.

◆ Adopt a city block or strip of road and keep it clean.

◆ Become a big brother or big sister at your local Boys & Girls Club.

◆ Help out at your local animal shelter.

◆ Train your pet and yourself to be a pet-therapy team.

◆ Become a docent at your local museum.

◆ Become a trail guide at a state or national park.

◆ Help out at your local hospital.

Volunteering can be a family affair, too. Many of the previously mentioned suggestions allow for children to pitch in as well. Find out about specific opportunities in your area by visiting www.volunteermatch.org. All you do is type in your zip code and your interests and—voilà!—a list of organizations and hot links to contact them appears. You can also go to charity.com for a list of over 200 worthy organizations.

Improve Your Own Neighborhood

A classic example of individuals coming together for a common purpose in order to serve others is the story of Tupelo, Mississippi. A newspaperman named George McLean took it upon himself, at the end of the 1930s, to turn around the economy of the town, which was dire at that time. He got local business owners to invest in the purchase of a costly high-quality stud bull. It launched a local dairy industry that turned the town around, benefiting everyone.

Seek out opportunities in your own neighborhood. Take a walk around the block. Go to the nearest playground. Think about what is needed. There are exciting and useful projects that are inaugurated every day by people just like you.

How Many Candles?

This Boston-born man earns a modest living from the small publishing house he owns in a small southern city. He is married with two grown sons and three grandchildren and two brothers. His relationship with his wife is solid (significant other AQ 43) and he is a very strong family man (family AQ 61). Healthy and fit (medical AQ 33, physical fitness AQ 29), he is extremely satisfied with his career and believes that his publishing house will continue to grow (financial AQ 46). He has a sterling community AQ of 66: he always votes, is very interested in politics and the issues of the day, gets his information from a variety of sources, attends community events at least once a month, and volunteers at least twice monthly. His self-image AQ is strong (71) as is his future AQ of 79: he is constantly educating himself, and keeps up with technology, which he finds exciting. He is very happy with his current situation, and, while he wouldn't switch careers, if challenging opportunities opened up elsewhere, he'd be willing to pull up stakes and move. His chronological age is 54; his true age: 56. A good example of a healthy, well-balanced, mature individual.

Engage in Politics

You may have a dozen and one excuses to stay away from the political arena. "They don't play fair." "You can't fight City Hall." "I can't make a difference, so why try?" "I don't want to be involved in politics!"

You can leave it up to everyone else. Just hope that you agree with them. But, as acclaimed anthropologist Margaret Mead once said, "Never doubt that a small group of thoughtful, committed citizens can change the world; indeed, it's the only thing that ever does." If you want to feel empowered, to feel a part of the fabric that makes up your life, you really can't avoid politics—its influence is too far reaching. Why not empower yourself and your family? Become a viable thread in the tapestry of your life.

It isn't only Washington, D.C. that's "by the people, of the people, and for the people." It's the community you live in, too. And on the local level, there are many things you can do. The simplest thing is to vote!

Here are some other ways:

- Write letters to the editor of your local paper.
- Make phone calls or pass out flyers for the political candidate of your choice.
- Join peaceful demonstrations that reflect your point of view.
- Join political organizations compatible with your views.

Even if you can't get out and do the things you believe in, you can spend some time in front of the computer as an armchair activist. Subscribe to the websites that reflect your values and attitudes. Sign their petitions. Distribute their announcements. Donate what you can.

Keep Up with Culture

The clothes you wear, the music you listen to, the films you attend, the books you read, the food you consume, the things you talk about, the way in which you relate to the fast-changing world around you—be it new technology or new art forms, alternative lifestyles or scientific discoveries—all have a great deal to do with your level of maturity as members of your community.

It's one thing for teenagers or very young adults to spend a lot of time and money keeping up with the almost-monthly changes in the fashion world, hanging out at the mall and saving up for the latest sports shoe. But the more mature adult will eventually formulate a style suitable to his or her own temperament and body type, rather than simply donning the latest and greatest in fun threads. As with all else, there is a balance to maintain.

How Many Candles?

Twice divorced, this teacher adopted and raised a son on her own. She's fit as a fiddle; she practices tai chi chuan regularly (physical fitness AQ 33), with no medical concerns (medical AQ 32); and she's successful and quite happy in her work (financial AQ 53). While not religious, she nonetheless attends and is active with a Unitarian church, yet her spiritual AQ is only 50 because, despite her efforts, she does not get any solace from it. She's always lived in big cites; she loves new challenges and is always learning, yet would love to put aside ambition so she could relax and enjoy more (future AQ 65). Bilingual, she has developed many skills, from languages to playing piano to painting (brain AQ 30). Committed to community service (community AQ 62), she votes in all elections, contributes to causes, attends community events a couple of times a month, and occasionally gets involved in activist or charitable works. She is not particularly happy about being single (singleness AQ 34). Her true age is 53. Her chronological age is 66. The only thing lacking in this mature, healthy genarian is her lack of spiritual fulfillment.

An excellent path to broadening your horizons is to expand your knowledge of the world by getting information from outside the mainstream media. Read newspapers from someplace other than your city, state, or country! Discover points of view from the rest of the world. The Internet is a great way to accomplish that.

In today's world, keeping up with your culture means keeping up with world culture. In so doing, you will surely come up with a mature community AQ. By thinking globally and acting locally, you will, in political scientist Robert Putnam's words, be working toward "a sustained, broad-based social movement to restore civic virtue and civic participation in America."

The Least You Need to Know

◆ You have an obligation to fulfill your civic duties.

◆ Volunteering is rewarding and essential to a healthy community.

◆ Individuals can make a difference.

◆ Political engagement goes way beyond party politics.

◆ A mature community true age demands you learn about the world around you.

Appendix A

Glossary

aerobic   Involving or improving oxygen consumption by the body.

anaerobic   The ability to be without oxygen.

andropause   Sometimes referred to as male menopause, it is caused by a reduced production of certain hormones, like testosterone.

arteriosclerosis   A chronic disease in which thickening, hardening, and loss of elasticity of the arterial walls result in impaired blood circulation.

autonomic nervous system   The part of the vertebrate nervous system that regulates involuntary action, as of the intestines, heart, and glands. It is divided into the sympathetic nervous system and the parasympathetic nervous system.

biofeedback   Method for learning to increase one's ability to control biological responses, such as blood pressure, muscle tension, and heart rate. Sophisticated instruments are often used to measure physiological responses and make them apparent to the patient, who then tries to alter and ultimately control them without the aid of monitoring devices.

biotechnology   The use of microorganisms, such as bacteria or yeasts, or biological substances, such as enzymes, to perform specific industrial or manufacturing processes.

cardiovascular   Relating to or involving the heart and the blood vessels. Cardiovascular diseases include angina, claudication, and high blood pressure (hypertension).

centenarian   One who has lived 100 years or more.

cerebral cortex   The extensive outer layer of gray matter of the cerebral hemispheres, largely responsible for higher brain functions, including sensation, voluntary muscle movement, thought, reasoning, and memory.

decrepitude   The quality or condition of being weakened, worn out, impaired, or broken down by old age, illness, or hard use.

diastolic   The normal, rhythmic period of time when the heart relaxes after contraction, during which it fills with blood.

dopamine   A hormone and neurotransmitter occurring in a wide variety of animals, including both vertebrates and invertebrates. It is commonly associated with the pleasure system of the brain.

dura or **dura mater**   The dura mater (Latin for "hard mother") is the tough, fibrous membrane covering the brain and the spinal cord and lining the inner surface of the skull.

entrainment   To pull or draw along after itself; to carry in a current.

estriol   An estrogenic hormone found in the urine during pregnancy.

estrogen   Any of several steroid hormones produced chiefly by the ovaries. It is responsible for promoting estrus, and the development and maintenance of female secondary sex characteristics.

genarian   Columnist Jack Smith's term for anyone in his 60s or older.

gerontologist   A scientist who studies the biological, psychological, and sociological phenomena associated with ageing and old age.

gerontophobe   Authors' term for a person who is fearful of getting older.

gerontophobia   Authors' term for the fear of getting older.

hypertension   Elevated blood pressure resulting from an increase in the amount of blood pumped by the heart, or from increased resistance to the flow of blood through the small arterial blood vessels (arterioles).

isoflavone   A class of organic compounds and biomolecules related to bioflavonoids. They are also very strong antioxidants, and have been thought by many as useful in treating cancer.

lipoprotein   Any organic compound that is composed of both protein and fat.

mirroring   In its simplest form, reflecting very closely through your reactions the state of mind of the other person (what she is thinking, feeling, doing). Such reactions are expressed via similar posture, gesture, facial expression, or tone of voice.

neuron   Also called a nerve cell, neurons are the core components of the brain and spinal cord. Each consists of a cell body with one or more dendrites and a single axon.

nonagenarian   A person in her 90s.

octogenarian   A person in his 80s.

orthostatic   The ability of the body to make sudden changes in posture.

osteoporosis   A disease in which the bones become extremely porous, are subject to fracture, and heal slowly. It occurs especially in women following menopause, often leading to curvature of the spine from vertebral collapse.

oxytocin   A hormone that stimulates the contraction of smooth muscle of the uterus during labor, and facilitates ejection of milk from the breast during nursing. In humans, oxytocin is thought to be released during hugging, touching, and orgasm in both sexes. In the brain, oxytocin is involved in social recognition and bonding, and may be involved in the formation of generosity and trust between people.

para amino benzoic acid (PABA)   Part of the vitamin B complex, it is an essential nutrient for some. However, PABA is not essential to human health, and is therefore not officially classified as a vitamin. It has been widely used in sunscreens to filter out ultraviolet light, although there is some controversy as to whether it may actually increase the risk of skin cancer.

pranayama   Sanskrit word meaning "lengthening of the prana or breath." Essential in all yogic practices, it is considered to be the science of energy control.

septuagenarian   A person in his 70s.

serotonin   Plays an important role as a neurotransmitter, in the inhibition of anger, aggression, body temperature, learning, mood, sleep, vomiting, sexuality, and appetite. Commonly used in antidepressant drugs.

sexagenarian   A person in her 60s.

synapse   The junction at which communication of nerve cells with one another takes place as they pass through axons and dendrites, converting electrical impulses into chemical signals.

systolic   The normal, rhythmic contraction of the heart, by which blood is driven through the aorta and pulmonary artery.

trans fat   A type of artificially hydrogenated fat that may be monounsaturated or polyunsaturated; it is industrially created for the purpose of extending shelf life.

transcendental meditation   A technique of meditation derived from Hindu traditions that promotes deep relaxation through the use of a mantra, which is a sacred verbal formula repeated in prayer or meditation.

triglycerides   Fats and oils that, in humans, supply fuel for energy. They are normally obtained from foods, but excessive sugar and alcohol consumption can cause them to be synthesized in the body. Elevated levels of triglycerides in the blood are associated with an increased risk of heart disease.

vasopressin   A hormone that regulates the body's retention of water and raises blood pressure. It is thought to be released into the brain during sexual activity, acting to initiate and sustain pair-bonding between the sexual partners.

Appendix B

Recommended Resources

Books

Ageing: The Great Adventure—A Buddhist Guide by Ken Jones (Aberystwyth, Wales: Pilgrim Press, 2003)

Aging and Time: Multidisciplinary Perspectives, Edited by J. Bars and H. Visser (Amityville, NY: Baywood Pub., 2007)

Aging Well by George E. Vaillant, M.D. (New York: Little, Browne & Co., 2002)

Breaking the Age Barrier by Elaine Partnow (Los Angeles: Pinnacle Books, 1981)

Breaking the Rules of Aging by David A. Lipschitz, M.D., Ph.D. (Washington, D.C.: Lifeline Press, 2002)

Changing Course: Navigating Life After 50 by William Sadler, Ph.D., and James Krefft, Ph.D. (The Center for Third Age Leadership Press, 2008)

Claiming Your Place at the Fire by Richard J. Leider and David A. Shapiro (San Francisco: Berrett-Koehler Publishers, 2004)

Ending Aging by Aubrey De Grey, Ph.D. (New York: St. Martin's Press, 2007)

The Fountain of Age by Betty Friedan (New York: Simon & Schuster, 1993)

Frames of Mind, The Theory of Multiple Intelligences by Howard Gardner (New York: BasicBooks, 1983)

From Age-ing to Sage-ing by Zalman Schachter-Shalomi and Ronald S. Miller (New York: Warner Books, 1995)

Getting Over Getting Older by Letty Cottin Pogrebin (New York: Little, Brown, 1996)

Journeying East: Conversations of Aging and Dying by Victoria Dimidjian (Berkeley, CA: Parallax Press, 2004)

The Life Extension Revolution by Philip Lee Miller, M.D. (New York: Bantam Books, 2005)

Living Without Regret: Growing Old in the Light of Tibetan Buddhism by Arnaud Maitland (Berkeley, CA: Dharma Pub., 2005)

Moving Toward Spiritual Maturity: Psychological, Contemplative, and Moral Challenges in Christian Living by Neil Pembroke (New York: Haworth Pastoral Press, 2007)

Successful Aging by John W. Rowe, M.D. and Robert L. Kahn, Ph.D. (New York City: Dell Publishing, 1998)

What Are Old People For? How Elders Will Save the World by William H. Thomas, M.D. (Acton, MA: VanderWyk & Burnham, 2004)

Websites

To further aide you, we've arranged these in three parts, correlating to the physical age quotients, inner workings, and the world around us.

Physical AQ Resources

American Academy of Anti-Aging Medicine (A4M)
www.worldhealth.net

Excellent health-related, anti-aging information.

American Association for Health Freedom
www.healthfreedom.net

The AAHF promote causes of health and well-being. The Association offers a search mechanism for finding a physician in your area.

American Society on Aging (ASA)
www.asaging.org

The ASA Forum on Religion, Spirituality, and Aging is highly informative and includes inspiring bibliographies and resources.

Better Ideal Weight Body Calculations
www.halls.md/ideal-weight/body.htm

Enter your weight, height, age, and gender, and it will calculate your ideal weight!

Council on Alcoholism and Treatment
www.aca-usa.org

Excellent information on drinking habits, alcohol abuse, and alcoholism.

Institute of HeartMath®
www.heartmath.org

Resources on the connections between the mind and heart.

The Methuselah Foundation
www.methuselahfoundation.org

Their motto is to "repair and reverse the damage of aging." Lots of interesting articles and blogs on life extension.

National Heart, Lung & Blood Institute
www.nhlbisupport.com/bmi

Has a free body mass index (BMI) calculator; just enter your height and weight.

Real Age
www.RealAge.com

Purportedly determines your biological age. It's fun to take (about 15 minutes). At its conclusion, it shows a column detailing what makes you younger, and another detailing what makes you older.

Revolution

www.revolutionhealth.com

Calling itself "your home for health and balance," it is a fount of sensible information on everything from diet to exercise, from diseases to food supplements. If you register, its interactive calculators enable you to follow various regimes—and it's free!

Spa Week

www.SpaWeek.org

A great source for discovering healing retreats near you. Registration is free. In 2008, they anticipate having over 500 participating day spas and 35–75 overnight retreats.

Inner Workings Resources

The Chopra Center

www.chopra.com

Deepak Chopra, the world-renowned Indian medical doctor and spiritual leader, has a website with a similar focus to Dr. Weil's, below, adding meditation and Ayurvedic medicines to its roster of well-being techniques.

Dr. Andrew Weil

www.drweil.com

The well-known physician/author focuses on healthy lifestyles, spirit and inspiration, supplements, and even pet care!

Dr. Michael Brickey's Ageless Lifestyles Institute

www.drbrickey.com/ageless-lifestyles-institute.htm

Lots of information for increasing longevity and helping people live longer, healthier, and happier lives.

SAGE-ING GUILD

www.sage-ingguild.org

A networking organization for professionals trained in the Sage-ing philosophy of Rabbi Zalman Schachter-Shalomi. Members of the Guild lead discussions, classes, and workshops designed for people interested in aging consciously and with purpose.

The World Around Us Resources

Career Explorer

www.careerexplorer.net

Career Success Training

www.careersuccesstraining.com

Quintessential Careers

www.quintcareers.com

If you're looking for new career possibilities, check out the preceding three websites.

Educational and Training Facilities

www.careerexplorer.net

Plug in the field that interests you along with your zip code and you will be led to campuses in your area as well as online programs in your field.

Resumé Writing

www.how-to-write-a-resume.org
www.howtowritearesume.net

Guidelines for putting together a professional resumé.

Volunteer Opportunities

www.volunteermatch.org
www.charity.com

Type in your zip code and interests on the first website and you'll get a list of local opportunities. The second site offers links to over 200 worthy charities.

Working Mother Magazine

www.workingmother.com

Lists the top-100 family-friendly corporations.

Index

Q

R

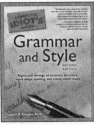
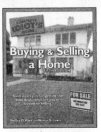
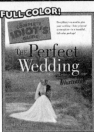
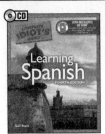
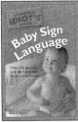
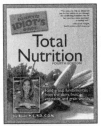
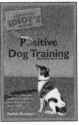
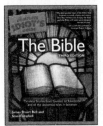
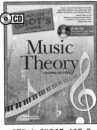
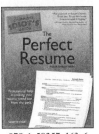
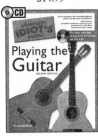
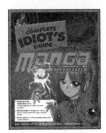
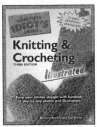
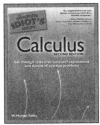
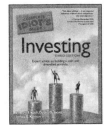